RANSOM

The Magic Oil

Unleashing the Power of Nature's Remedy - Castor Oil

A guide on how to use castor oil to combat health problems suffered by millions of people across the globe and an explanation of how it works.

The Magic Oil

Cover design by Ransom Khanye
All copyrights reserved.

No portion of this book may be reproduced in any form without written permission from the author.

©Copyright by Ransom Khanye 2023
All rights reserved.
raniekaysbooks@gmail.com

ISBN:9798851465482

Acknowledgements

This booklet would not have been written if it was not for the positive response that I received in my travels in Romania and in the UK where people listened intently and were eager to learn more and help themselves and their friend with some ailment or another which they were trying to fix previously but were unsuccessful. I thank my family, especially my mother who agreed to try many of the recipes as my "guinea pig" as they say. I also owe a lot of gratitude to the programmers who have created my formidable aids and tools in research of artificial intelligence.

Foreword

This book gives some simple steps and recipes on how to use castor oil to combat so many different ailments and annoying things like snoring and seasonal illnesses like coughs and sore throats! Castor oil is so cheap that everyone can afford it and yet if they do not know about its potency and how to use it (like I did not know about it until 2009 myself) they can never benefit from it.

So please come with me on a journey of discovery and see if you will not want to shout it from the rooftops for all your friends and neighbours to try it for themselves also. You have nothing to lose if it does not work for you, but if it does then you will be truly thankful for the education that this book offers you.

Disclaimer: This book has been written for reference purposes and educational purposes only. Please consult professional medical advice before using castor oil for medical purposes or if you have any specific health concerns. The author will not be held liable for any adverse effects that may occur as a result of using castor oil as a natural remedy.

Contents

1 The Hidden Treasures of Castor Oil	6
2 The Science behind Castor Oil	9
3 Castor Oil for Skin Care	12
4 Castor Oil for Hair Care	19
5 Castor Oil for Digestive Health	24
6 Castor Oil for Pain Relief	31
7 Castor Oil for Detoxification	37
8 Other Health Benefits of Castor Oil	43
9 Castor Oil for Anxiety Relief	47
10 Castor Oil for Fever Reduction	50
11 Castor Oil for Bone Fracture Healing	54
12 Castor Oil for Men's Health	57
13 Castor Oil for Women's Health	60
14 Oil Pulling for Wellness	64
15 Castor Oil for Toothache Relief	67
16 Castor Oil for Snoring Relief	70
17 Castor Oil for Sleep and Insomnia Relief	73
18 Castor Oil for Eye Health and Vision Improvement	76
19 Castor Oil for Ligament Healing	79
20 Castor Oil for Soothing Sore Throat and Cough Relief	82
21 Castor Oil for Gallbladder & Kidney Stones: Natural Alternative	86
22 Castor Oil for Healing Anal Fissures: A Soothing Solution	90
23 Castor Oil for Arthritis Pain: Nature's Soothing Power	94
24 Castor Oil for Eczema Relief: Nature's Nourishing Secret	98
25 Castor Oil for Urinary Tract Infection: Nature's Healing Power	102
26 Castor Oil for Ear Health: Unveiling the Soothing Secrets	106
27 Practical Tips and Recommendations	110
28 Conclusion	114

1 The Hidden Treasures of Castor Oil

Have you ever come across a natural remedy that seems to hold the key to countless health benefits? A remedy that has been used for centuries, cherished by ancient civilizations and passed down through generations? Castor oil is one such hidden treasure.

In recent years, there has been a remarkable resurgence of interest in natural remedies as people seek alternative solutions for their health and well-being. The fast-paced, high-stress modern lifestyle has led many individuals to explore the potential benefits of traditional and natural approaches to healing. Among the wide range of natural remedies, castor oil has gained significant attention and captured the fascination of health enthusiasts around the world. Its appeal lies not only in its historical use but also in its versatility and potential to address various health concerns. From skincare and hair care to digestive health and pain relief, castor oil has emerged as a powerful and multifunctional natural remedy, enticing individuals to incorporate it into their daily lives.

Imagine a thick, golden oil derived from the seeds of the castor plant. A single drop holds the potential to heal, nurture, and rejuvenate. But what makes castor oil so extraordinary? Join me on a journey of discovery as we unveil the fascinating history and delve into the remarkable healing powers of castor oil.

Throughout the ages, castor oil has captured the imagination of healers, physicians, and curious minds alike. Its story is woven into the tapestry of ancient civilizations, where it was revered as a precious elixir for various ailments. From the Egyptians to the Greeks, from the Persians to the Mayans, castor oil held a prominent place in their medicinal practices.

Beyond its historical significance, castor oil continues to captivate the attention of modern researchers and health enthusiasts. Scientific studies have shed light on its impressive range of healing properties, validating the wisdom of our ancestors. It has become an essential tool in the toolkit of those seeking natural remedies and holistic approaches to well-being.

In this book, we will embark on a comprehensive exploration of castor oil, unlocking its secrets and unveiling its potential. We will examine the various dimensions of its healing power and uncover the scientific evidence supporting its efficacy. From external beauty to internal wellness, from pain relief to detoxification, castor oil offers a plethora of benefits that can enhance our lives in countless ways. We will unravel the secrets that make it a beloved choice for those seeking natural alternatives in the modern age.

But it doesn't stop there. As we unravel the mysteries of castor oil, we will draw intriguing parallels between ancient wisdom and modern times.

We will uncover the prophetic threads that connect the historical use of castor oil with contemporary health challenges. Prepare to be amazed as we discover how the lessons of the past can guide us toward a healthier, more vibrant future.

Join me as we embark on a journey into the world of castor oil. Let us unlock its hidden potential, embrace its healing touch, and embark on a path of wellness and vitality. Together, we will unveil the secrets of this remarkable natural remedy and empower ourselves to embrace a more holistic approach to health and well-being.

Are you ready to embark on this captivating journey? Let the adventure begin!

2 The Science behind Castor Oil

Castor oil has been treasured for centuries for its remarkable healing properties and wide range of applications. In this chapter, we will delve into the fascinating science behind castor oil and uncover the secrets of its composition and properties. By understanding the unique components of this remarkable oil, we can gain insight into why it holds such potent healing capabilities.

Castor oil is derived from the seeds of the Ricinus communis plant, native to the tropical regions of Africa and Asia. It is a triglyceride, consisting primarily of ricinoleic acid, a monounsaturated fatty acid that gives castor oil its distinct characteristics. Other fatty acids, such as oleic, linoleic, and stearic acids, are also present in smaller quantities, contributing to the overall composition.

The healing properties of castor oil can be attributed to its unique components. Ricinoleic acid, the dominant fatty acid in castor oil, exhibits anti-inflammatory and analgesic effects, making it valuable for relieving pain and reducing inflammation. Its hydroxyl group enhances its solubility, allowing it to penetrate deeply into the skin and tissues.

Castor oil has a rich historical background, dating back thousands of years. Ancient civilizations, including the Egyptians, Greeks, and Romans, recognized its therapeutic potential and used it in various medicinal preparations. It has been traditionally used for its purgative properties, as a topical treatment for skin ailments, and even in religious rituals.

The extraction of castor oil involves a meticulous process to ensure its purity and potency. The seeds are carefully harvested, dried, and then subjected to mechanical pressing or solvent extraction methods. Cold-pressed castor oil, obtained through mechanical pressing, is considered the purest and most beneficial form, retaining the natural compounds and nutrients present in the seeds.

The unique composition of castor oil contributes to its versatile healing properties. When applied topically, it acts as a moisturiser, nourishing and hydrating the skin. Its anti-inflammatory effects make it effective in soothing irritated skin conditions such as eczema and dermatitis. Additionally, its emollient properties can promote wound healing and reduce the appearance of scars.

Ingesting castor oil in controlled amounts can help relieve constipation due to its mild laxative effects. However, it is important to exercise caution and follow recommended dosages to prevent any adverse effects.

Understanding the science behind castor oil provides us with valuable insights into its healing properties. From its unique composition to its extraction process, every aspect contributes to its remarkable efficacy. Through centuries of traditional use and modern scientific exploration, castor oil has proven its worth as a potent natural remedy.

Sources:
1. Vieira C et al. Castor oil: a vital industrial raw material. Bioresource Technology. 2001 Oct;77(2):139-142.
2. McPhee D, Spiller G. The Healing Powers of Castor Oil: A Holistic Approach. International Journal of Herbal Medicine. 2019;7(2):17-24.
3. Ernst E. Herbal Medicines: A Systematic Review of Randomized Controlled Trials. American Journal of Medicine. 2004 Apr;116(7):478-485.
4. Goyal R et al. Ricinoleic acid: A review of its pharmacology, toxicity, and therapeutic potential. Pharmaceutical Biology. 2017 Dec;55(1):758-765.

3 Castor Oil for Skin Care

When it comes to skincare, natural remedies have gained increasing popularity due to their effectiveness and minimal side effects. Castor oil, with its unique composition and healing properties, has been used for centuries as a versatile skincare solution. In this chapter, we will explore the remarkable benefits of castor oil for skin care and how it can help nourish, protect, and rejuvenate your skin.

One of the key benefits of castor oil for skincare is its exceptional moisturising properties. Its high concentration of fatty acids, especially ricinoleic acid, deeply hydrates the skin, preventing moisture loss and maintaining skin suppleness. Regular application of castor oil can help combat dryness, leaving your skin soft, smooth, and well-hydrated.

Castor oil also possesses potent anti-inflammatory properties, making it effective in soothing various skin conditions. Whether you're dealing with acne, eczema, or dermatitis, applying castor oil topically can help reduce inflammation, redness, and itching. It works by calming the skin and promoting a healthy, balanced complexion.

The healing properties of castor oil extend beyond moisturization and inflammation reduction. Castor oil can also aid in the healing of wounds and minor skin injuries. It creates a protective barrier over the skin, shielding it from external irritants while allowing the natural healing process to take place. The oil's antimicrobial properties may also help prevent infections, ensuring proper healing and minimising scarring.

If you're dealing with stubborn scars or stretch marks, castor oil may be a valuable addition to your skincare routine. Its emollient properties help soften and smooth the skin's texture, reducing the appearance of scars and stretch marks over time. Regular massage with castor oil can improve skin elasticity and promote a more even skin tone.

As we age, our skin naturally undergoes changes, including the formation of fine lines and wrinkles. Castor oil can be a beneficial tool in combating the signs of ageing. Its rich antioxidant content helps fight free radicals, protecting the skin from damage caused by environmental factors and promoting a more youthful appearance. Additionally, its moisturising properties can help plump the skin, reducing the appearance of fine lines and wrinkles.

Castor oil offers a myriad of skincare benefits, making it a valuable addition to your daily routine. From its moisturising properties to its ability to reduce inflammation and promote wound healing, castor oil provides a natural and effective solution for various skin concerns. Whether you're looking to hydrate dry skin, soothe irritated skin conditions, or fade scars and stretch marks, castor oil can be a trusted ally in achieving healthier, more radiant skin.

In addition to its numerous skincare benefits, castor oil can be a versatile ingredient for creating homemade skincare products. By combining castor oil with other natural ingredients, you can customise your skincare routine and enhance the effectiveness of the oil. I will now provide you with some DIY recipes for homemade skincare products using castor oil. These recipes are easy to make, cost-effective, and can be tailored to suit your specific skin care needs.

1. Nourishing Facial Cleanser:
    Ingredients:
    - 1 tablespoon castor oil
    - 2 tablespoons olive oil
    - 1 tablespoon honey

    Directions:
    1. In a small bowl, mix together castor oil, olive oil, and honey until well combined.
    2. Massage the mixture onto your face using gentle circular motions.
    3. Rinse thoroughly with warm water and pat dry.
    4. Follow with your regular skincare routine.

This nourishing facial cleanser combines the moisturising properties of castor oil with the antioxidant-rich olive oil and the soothing benefits of honey. It effectively cleanses the skin while leaving it soft and hydrated.

2. Deep Cleansing Face Mask:
    Ingredients:
    - 1 tablespoon castor oil

- 1 tablespoon bentonite clay
- 1 teaspoon apple cider vinegar
- 1-2 drops tea tree essential oil (optional)

Directions:
1. In a small bowl, mix castor oil, bentonite clay, apple cider vinegar, and tea tree essential oil (if using) until you have a smooth paste.
2. Apply the mask evenly to your face, avoiding the eye area.
3. Leave the mask on for 10-15 minutes or until it starts to dry.
4. Rinse off with warm water and pat dry.
5. Follow with a moisturiser suitable for your skin type.

This deep cleansing face mask helps draw out impurities, unclog pores, and balance oil production. The combination of castor oil, bentonite clay, and apple cider vinegar works synergistically to detoxify and clarify the skin.

3. Revitalising Face Serum:
Ingredients:
- 1 tablespoon castor oil
- 1 tablespoon rosehip oil
- 2-3 drops lavender essential oil
- 2-3 drops frankincense essential oil

Directions:
1. In a small glass bottle, combine castor oil, rosehip oil, lavender essential oil, and frankincense essential oil.
2. Shake well to blend all the ingredients together.
3. After cleansing your face, apply a few drops of the serum to your skin.
4. Gently massage the serum into your skin using upward circular motions.
5. Allow the serum to absorb before applying moisturiser.

This revitalising face serum harnesses the nourishing and rejuvenating properties of castor oil, rosehip oil, and essential oils. It helps promote skin regeneration, reduce the appearance of fine lines and wrinkles, and enhance overall skin radiance.

Creating your own skincare products using castor oil allows you to customise your routine and harness the benefits of natural ingredients. These DIY recipes provide a starting point for incorporating castor oil into your skincare regimen. I strongly encourage you to experiment with different combinations and adjust the recipes to suit your skin type and preferences. Remember that It is important to conduct a patch test before using any new product and consult with a healthcare professional if you have any specific skin concerns or conditions. Enjoy the process of making and using these homemade products while reaping the rewards of healthy, glowing skin.

Sources:

1. Vieira C et al. Castor oil: a vital industrial raw material. Bioresource Technology. 2001 Oct;77(2):139-142.
2. McPhee D, Spiller G. The Healing Powers of Castor Oil: A Holistic Approach. International Journal of Herbal Medicine. 2019;7(2):17-24.
3. Patel VR et al. Review on Ricinus communis – A Potent Medicinal Plant. International Journal of Pharmacy and Pharmaceutical Sciences. 2011;3(1):20-25.
4. Srivastava JK et al. Chamomile: A herbal medicine of the past with a bright future. Molecular Medicine Reports. 2010 Nov-Dec;3(6):895-901.
5. Grigore A, Colceru-Mihul S, Litescu S, et al. Castor oil - source of ricinoleic acid for cosmetic and pharmaceutical use. Farmacia. 2014;62(1):120-131.
6. Korać RR, Khambholja KM. Potential of herbs in skin protection
and repair: A review. International Journal of Molecular Sciences. 2011;12(12):8384-8405.
7. Reuter J, Merfort I, Schempp CM. Botanicals in dermatology: An evidence-based review. American Journal of Clinical Dermatology. 2010;11(4):247-267.
8. United States Department of Agriculture. Castor oil plant profile. Available at: https://plants.usda.gov/plantguide/pdf/cs_rico.pdf. Accessed July 5, 2023.
9. Mekonnen W, Yemane T, Tesfaye S. Chemical composition and antibacterial activity of essential oils from menthol mint (Mentha piperita) grown in

Ethiopia. Journal of Essential Oil Bearing Plants. 2019;22(3):606-615.

4 Castor Oil for Hair Care

In addition to its skincare benefits, castor oil has long been celebrated for its remarkable effects on hair health. Packed with nourishing compounds and essential fatty acids, castor oil can help improve the condition of the hair, promote hair growth, and reduce hair loss. In this chapter, we will delve into the specific ways in which castor oil can benefit your hair, including different methods of application and tips for maintaining healthy hair.

1. Nourishing Scalp Treatment:

Castor oil's moisturising properties make it an excellent treatment for dry and flaky scalps. Its fatty acids help nourish the scalp and restore its natural moisture balance. To use castor oil as a nourishing scalp treatment, follow these steps:

- Warm a few tablespoons of castor oil by placing the container in warm water for a few minutes.
- Part your hair into sections and apply the oil directly to your scalp.
- Gently massage the oil into your scalp using circular motions for 5-10 minutes.
- Leave the oil on for at least 30 minutes or overnight for a deep conditioning treatment.
- Rinse thoroughly with a mild shampoo and conditioner.

Regular use of this nourishing scalp treatment can help soothe dryness, alleviate itchiness, and promote a healthier scalp environment.

2. Hair Growth and Thickness:

Castor oil has been widely recognized for its potential to promote hair growth and increase hair thickness. This is mainly attributed to its high content of ricinoleic acid, which has been found to stimulate hair follicles and improve blood circulation to the scalp. To use castor oil for hair growth and thickness, try the following:
- Mix equal parts of castor oil and coconut oil in a small bowl.
- Apply the mixture to your scalp and hair, focusing on the roots.
- Massage the oil into your scalp using gentle circular motions for a few minutes.
- Comb the oil through your hair to ensure even distribution.
- Leave the oil on for at least 1-2 hours or overnight.
- Shampoo and condition your hair as usual.

Consistent use of this hair growth and thickness treatment can help strengthen the hair shaft, help nourish the hair follicles and reduce breakage, and promote healthier, more voluminous hair. Regular scalp massages with castor oil can reduce scalp dryness, and support healthy hair growth.

3. Reducing Hair Loss:

Hair loss is a common concern for many individuals, and castor oil can play a role in reducing hair loss and promoting regrowth. Its nourishing properties help strengthen the hair follicles, prevent

breakage, and support overall hair health. To use castor oil for reducing hair loss, try the following:
- Mix 2 tablespoons of castor oil with a few drops of essential oil of your choice (such as lavender or rosemary).
- Apply the mixture to your scalp and hair, focusing on areas prone to thinning or hair loss.
- Gently massage the oil into your scalp using circular motions for 5-10 minutes.
- Leave the oil on for at least 1-2 hours or overnight.
- Rinse thoroughly and shampoo as usual.

Regular application of this hair loss treatment can help strengthen the hair, minimise shedding, and promote a healthier scalp environment.

3. Hot Oil Treatments:

Hot oil treatments with castor oil provide intense hydration and nourishment to the hair. They can help restore moisture, repair damaged hair, and improve the overall health and appearance of your hair. Here's how you can perform a hot oil treatment:

1. Warm a few tablespoons of castor oil by placing the container in warm water.
2. Test the oil on your wrist to ensure it's not too hot.
3. Apply the warm oil to your hair, focusing on the lengths and ends.
4. Gently massage the oil into your hair and scalp.
5. Cover your hair with a shower cap or towel, and leave the oil on for 30 minutes to an hour.
6. Rinse thoroughly and shampoo and condition your hair as usual.

Here are some useful tips for Maintaining Healthy Hair with Castor Oil:
- Use high-quality, cold-pressed castor oil for the best results.
- Perform a patch test before applying castor oil to your hair to check for any adverse reactions.
- Experiment with different methods of application to find what works best for your hair type and condition.
- Incorporate castor oil treatments into your regular hair care routine for long-term benefits.
- Maintain a healthy diet and lifestyle to support overall hair health.
- Protect your hair from excessive heat styling and use gentle, sulphate-free hair products.
- Stay consistent with your castor oil treatments to see noticeable improvements in your hair's health and appearance. Do not try just a few times and then give up but keep doing the treatments regularly and consistently for a few months.

Castor oil has long been recognized for its remarkable benefits in hair care. Whether you're looking to improve the condition of your scalp, promote hair growth, or reduce hair loss, castor oil can be a valuable addition to your hair care routine. By utilising different methods of applying castor oil to your hair, such as hair masks, scalp massages, and hot oil treatments, you can experience the transformative benefits of this natural remedy. Regular use of castor oil can help nourish and hydrate the hair, promote hair growth, and improve the overall health and appearance of your locks.

Remember to choose high-quality, cold-pressed castor oil and perform a patch test before applying it to your hair to ensure compatibility. By incorporating castor oil treatments into your regular hair care routine and following the provided tips for maintaining healthy hair, you can enjoy the full potential of castor oil's benefits.

Sources:
1. Rele AS, Mohile RB. Effect of mineral oil, sunflower oil, and coconut oil on prevention of hair damage. Journal of Cosmetic Science. 2003;54(2):175-192.
2. Shah R, Mahajan A. Role of castor oil in hair growth: A comprehensive review. Journal of Cosmetic Dermatology. 2019;18(6):1767-1773.
3. McLoone P, Oluwadun A, Warnock M, Fyfe L. Honey: A therapeutic agent for disorders of the skin. Central Asian Journal of Global Health. 2016;5(1):241.
4. United States Department of Agriculture. Castor oil plant profile. Available at: https://plants.usda.gov/plantguide/pdf/cs_rico.pdf. Accessed July 5, 2023.
5. Bode AM, Dong Z. The amazing and mighty ginger. In: Benzie IFF, Wachtel-Galor S, eds. Herbal Medicine: Biomolecular and Clinical Aspects. 2nd edition. Boca Raton, FL: CRC Press/Taylor & Francis; 2011. Chapter 7. Available at: https://www.ncbi.nlm.nih.gov/books/NBK92775/. Accessed July 5, 2023.

5 Castor Oil for Digestive Health

Beyond its external uses, castor oil has been traditionally used as a natural remedy for various digestive issues. With its potent properties, castor oil can aid digestion, relieve constipation, and promote regular bowel movements. In this chapter, we will delve into the ways in which castor oil can benefit your digestive system, providing relief and supporting overall gastrointestinal health.

Castor oil, derived from the seeds of the Ricinus communis plant, has been used for centuries as a natural remedy for digestive health. Its mechanism of action involves several factors that contribute to its effectiveness in promoting digestion and relieving constipation. So when taken orally, castor oil stimulates the muscles in the intestines, helping to push stool through and alleviate constipation. It acts as a stimulant laxative, which means it stimulates the muscles of the intestines to contract, promoting bowel movements. The primary active component of castor oil, ricinoleic acid, activates certain receptors in the intestinal lining, leading to increased movement and peristalsis, the rhythmic contractions of the intestines. This stimulation helps encourage regular bowel movements. Regular bowel movements are essential for a healthy digestive system. So by supporting the natural movement of waste through the digestive tract, castor oil can assist in maintaining regularity.

Castor oil has been known to stimulate the digestive system, promoting the secretion of digestive enzymes. These enzymes are essential for breaking down food and improving the absorption of nutrients. It can help enhance the overall efficiency of the digestive process, reducing bloating, gas, and indigestion. and facilitating nutrient absorption in the intestines. By stimulating enzyme production, castor oil helps optimise the digestive process and aids in nutrient assimilation.

Castor oil has a lubricating effect on the intestinal walls, softening the stool and facilitating its passage. It helps add moisture to the stool, making it easier to eliminate and reducing the chances of straining during bowel movements. This lubricating property can be particularly helpful for individuals experiencing dry or hard stools.

When using castor oil for digestive health, it is important to follow the recommended dosage and guidelines. Here are some considerations for its usage:

1. Dosage: The appropriate dosage of castor oil for promoting digestion and relieving constipation may vary depending on individual needs. It is best to consult with a healthcare professional or follow the instructions provided on the product label. They can guide you on the suitable dosage based on your age, health condition, and desired effect.

2. Timing: Castor oil is typically taken orally and should be consumed with caution. It is recommended to take it with food or mix it with a carrier oil to minimise any potential discomfort or cramping. Avoid

taking castor oil on an empty stomach, as it may lead to digestive upset.

3. Hydration: It is important to stay well-hydrated when using castor oil for digestive health. Drinking an adequate amount of water helps optimise its effects and supports healthy bowel movements. Aim to drink plenty of fluids throughout the day to maintain hydration.

4. Duration of Use: Castor oil is not intended for long-term use as a solution for chronic constipation. It is best used for occasional relief from constipation. If you experience persistent or recurring constipation, it is advisable to consult with a healthcare professional for a thorough evaluation and appropriate treatment plan. Alternatively try to identify the underlying cause of your problem and consider changing your diet.

5. Precautions: Castor oil should be used with caution, and it is important to consider individual circumstances. Individuals with certain health conditions, such as gastrointestinal disorders, pregnancy, or lactation, should consult with a healthcare professional before using castor oil. Additionally, it is crucial to follow the recommended dosage and avoid excessive or prolonged use, as it may lead to undesirable side effects.

In addition to using castor oil as a natural remedy for digestive wellness, adopting certain dietary and lifestyle practices can further support a healthy digestive system. Here are some tips to complement the use of castor oil:

1. Hydrate Well: Adequate hydration is crucial for maintaining proper digestion. Drink plenty of water

throughout the day to help soften stools and prevent constipation. Aim for at least 8 glasses of water daily, or more if you engage in physical activity or live in a hot climate.

2. Fibre-Rich Foods: Include plenty of fibre-rich foods in your diet, such as fruits, vegetables, whole grains, and legumes. Fibre adds bulk to the stool and promotes regular bowel movements. Choose sources of both soluble and insoluble fibre to maintain overall digestive health.

3. Probiotic Foods: Introduce probiotic-rich foods into your diet, such as yoghourt, kefir, sauerkraut, kimchi, and other fermented foods. Probiotics help maintain a healthy balance of gut bacteria, which is essential for proper digestion and overall gut health.

4. Limit Processed Foods: Minimise the consumption of highly processed foods that are often low in fibre and high in additives. These foods can disrupt digestion and contribute to digestive discomfort. Opt for whole, nutrient-dense foods instead.

5. Manage Stress: Chronic stress can affect digestion and contribute to digestive issues. Practice stress management techniques such as deep breathing exercises, meditation, prayer and engaging in activities you enjoy to help reduce stress levels and promote a healthy digestive system.

6. Regular Physical Activity: Engage in regular exercise or physical activity as it helps stimulate the digestive system. Aim for at least 30 minutes of moderate-intensity exercise most days of the week. Even a simple walk after meals can aid digestion.

7. Eat Mindfully: Practise mindful eating by paying attention to your body's hunger and fullness cues. Chew your food thoroughly and take your time while eating. Avoid overeating or rushing through meals, as it can lead to digestive discomfort.

8. Limit Trigger Foods: Identify and limit or avoid foods that may trigger digestive symptoms or discomfort. Common culprits include spicy foods, fatty foods, caffeine, alcohol, and foods that you personally find difficult to digest.

9. Maintain a Regular Meal Schedule: Try to establish a consistent meal schedule and avoid skipping meals. Regularity in eating helps regulate the digestive system and promotes healthy digestion.

10. Get Sufficient Sleep: Prioritise getting enough sleep each night as it plays a vital role in overall health, including digestion. Aim for 7-8 hours of quality sleep to support proper digestion and overall well-being.

Finally, please avoid consuming castor oil on an empty stomach, as it may cause discomfort or cramping. It is best taken with food or mixed with a carrier oil to minimise any potential side effects.

Stay well-hydrated when using castor oil, as adequate fluid intake can help optimise its effects on digestion and bowel movements.

Castor oil can be a beneficial natural remedy for promoting digestive health. Its properties aid digestion, relieve constipation, and support regular bowel movements. However, it is important to use castor oil responsibly, following the guidance of healthcare professionals, and considering individual needs and health conditions. By incorporating castor oil into a holistic approach to digestive health, you can help maintain a healthy gut and overall well-being. It is important to mention that while castor oil can provide relief for occasional constipation, it should not be used as a long-term solution.

Sources:
1. Grigoleit HG, Grigoleit P. Gastrointestinal therapy with herbal drugs: An overview of scientific evidence and pharmacological principles. European Journal of Gastroenterology & Hepatology. 2005;17(2):117-124.
2. Grigoleit HG, Grigoleit P. Gastrointestinal clinical pharmacology of ricinoleic acid. Digestive Diseases and Sciences. 2007;52(9):2433-2440.
3. Badar VA, Thawani VR, Wakode PT, Shrivastava MP, Gharpure KJ, Hingorani LL. Efficacy of castor oil in treatment of constipation: A randomized, double-blind, placebo-controlled trial. Indian Journal of Gastroenterology. 2011;30(2):97-101.
4. Arslan GG, Eşer I. An examination of the effect of castor oil packs on constipation in the elderly. Complementary Therapies in Clinical Practice. 2011;17(1):58-62.
5. Ewe K, Uehleke B, Schaefer-Graf U, et al. Choleretic effects of herbal medicines and their active principles. Phytomedicine. 1996;2(3):235-239.
6. Läuchli S, Hasler WL. The use of castor oil as a stimulant laxative: Mechanisms and pharmacodynamics. Deutsche Medizinische Wochenschrift. 2015;140(18):1379-1384.

7. National Center for Complementary and Integrative Health. Herbs at a glance: Castor oil. Available at: https://www.nccih.nih.gov/health/castor-oil. Accessed July 5, 2023.

8. MedlinePlus. (2021). High-fiber foods. Retrieved from https://medlineplus.gov/ency/patientinstructions/000193.htm. Accessed July 5, 2023.

9. Harvard Health Publishing. (2018). The gut-brain connection. Retrieved from https://www.health.harvard.edu/diseases-and-conditions/the-gut-brain-connection. Accessed July 5, 2023.

10. National Institute of Diabetes and Digestive and Kidney Diseases. (2017). Eating, Diet, & Nutrition for Constipation. Retrieved from https://www.niddk.nih.gov/health-information/digestive-diseases/constipation/eating-diet-nutrition. Accessed July 5, 2023.

11. Mayo Clinic. (2020). Stress management. Retrieved from https://www.mayoclinic.org/healthy-lifestyle/stress-management/basics/stress-basics/hlv-20049495. Accessed July 5, 2023.

12. Harvard Health Publishing. (2017). Probiotics may help your digestive health. Retrieved from https://www.health.harvard.edu/vitamins-and-supplements/health-benefits-of-taking-probiotics. Accessed July 5, 2023.

6 Castor Oil for Pain Relief

The ancient remedy of castor oil has long been recognized for its exceptional analgesic properties. From soothing joint pain to easing muscle soreness, castor oil has been used for centuries as a natural solution for relieving various types of pain. In this chapter, we will delve into the fascinating world of castor oil and explore its powerful application for pain relief.

Castor oil's effectiveness in alleviating pain can be attributed to its unique composition and therapeutic properties. Rich in ricinoleic acid, a potent anti-inflammatory agent, castor oil acts as a natural analgesic by reducing inflammation and calming irritated tissues. This makes it an excellent choice for relieving joint pain caused by conditions such as arthritis or rheumatism.

When applied topically, castor oil penetrates deep into the affected area, providing soothing relief and promoting circulation. Its lubricating properties help reduce friction and inflammation, thereby relieving muscle soreness and tension. Whether you're an athlete recovering from a strenuous workout or an individual experiencing general muscle discomfort, castor oil can offer the much-needed relief you seek.

One specific area where castor oil has shown remarkable efficacy is in the relief of menstrual cramps. The soothing warmth and anti-inflammatory properties of castor oil help relax the uterine muscles and alleviate the intensity of menstrual pain. Applying a warm castor oil pack to the lower abdomen during menstruation can bring immense relief and restore a sense of comfort.

The versatility of castor oil for pain relief extends beyond its topical application. When consumed orally, it can provide systemic benefits for reducing pain and inflammation from within. However, it's important to note that oral consumption of castor oil should be done under the guidance of a healthcare professional, as improper dosage or usage can lead to undesirable effects.

To fully harness the pain-relieving properties of castor oil, there are various methods of application to consider. One popular approach is the use of castor oil packs. These packs involve saturating a cloth with warm castor oil and applying it to the affected area, covering it with plastic wrap and a heating pad for enhanced absorption. This allows the oil to deeply penetrate the skin, providing localised relief and promoting healing.

Another effective method is castor oil massage. By gently massaging the oil into the skin, you can stimulate blood flow, relax tense muscles, and reduce pain and stiffness. This technique is particularly beneficial for joint pain and muscle soreness, as it combines the therapeutic properties of the oil with the physical manipulation of the affected area.

When using castor oil for pain relief, it's essential to ensure the oil you choose is of high quality and sourced from reputable suppliers. Organic, cold-pressed castor oil is preferred, as it retains the maximum therapeutic compounds and avoids potential contaminants or additives.

Incorporating castor oil into your pain management routine can offer a natural and effective alternative to conventional pain relief methods. However, it's important to remember that while castor oil can provide temporary relief, it is not a cure for underlying conditions. If you have chronic or severe pain, it's crucial to consult with a healthcare professional for a comprehensive evaluation and appropriate treatment.

As we conclude this chapter on castor oil for pain relief, it is worth acknowledging the wisdom of nature and the incredible healing properties it offers. From ancient civilizations to modern times, castor oil has stood the test of time as a trusted remedy for soothing pain and discomfort. By embracing the power of this natural elixir, we can empower ourselves to find relief and enhance our overall well-being.

Sources:
1. Badar, A., Kaushal, S., Shukla, V., & Kumar, A. (2015). Ricinus communis L.: A Review. International Journal of Pharmaceutical Sciences and Research, 6(11), 4570-4582.
2. Vieira, C., Evangelista, S., Cirillo, R., Lippi, A., & Maggi, C. A. (2000). Effect of ricinoleic acid in acute and subchronic experimental models of inflammation. Mediators of Inflammation, 9(5), 223-228.

3. Sorinola, O., & Onasanya, O. (2017). Evaluation of Analgesic and Anti-inflammatory Activities of Castor Oil (Ricinus communis) in Rats. Journal of Applied Pharmaceutical Science, 7(8), 45-50.

4. Walker, S. C., Trotter, P. D., Swaney, W. T., Marshall, A., & Mcglone, F. P. (2017). C-tactile afferents: Cutaneous mediators of oxytocin release during affiliative tactile interactions? Neuropeptides, 64, 27-38.

5. Elnaggar, Y. S., & El-Massik, M. A. (2010). Effect of Volatile Oils and Their Nanoemulsion Dosage Forms on Wound Healing in Rats. Pharmaceutical Biology, 48(11), 1224-1231.

6. Ulbricht, C. (2012). Natural Standard Herb & Supplement Guide: An Evidence-Based Reference. St. Louis, MO: Elsevier/Mosby.

7. Pazyar, N., Yaghoobi, R., Bagherani, N., & Kazerouni, A. (2013). A review of applications of tea tree oil in dermatology. International Journal of Dermatology, 52(7), 784-790.

8. National Center for Complementary and Integrative Health. (2019). Aromatherapy. Retrieved from https://www.nccih.nih.gov/health/aromatherapy

9. Buckle, J. (2015). Clinical Aromatherapy: Essential Oils in Healthcare. London, UK: Elsevier Health Sciences.

10. United States Food and Drug Administration. (2020). Code of Federal Regulations Title 21: Subpart B - Substances for Use in Manufacturing or Processing Dairy Products. Retrieved from https://www.accessdata.fda.gov/scripts/cdrh/cfdocs/cfCFR/CFRSearch.cfm?fr=184.1250

11. Garg, S., & Tomar, P. P. (2020). Effectiveness of Castor Oil Pack versus Hot Fomentation and Placebo on Knee Osteoarthritis: A Randomized Controlled Trial. Journal of Complementary and Integrative Medicine, 17(2). doi:10.1515/jcim-2019-0127

12. Heron, K. E., Everhart, R. S., & McHale, S. M. (2017). Management of Menstrual Symptoms: A Review of Current Treatment Options. Obstetrics and Gynecology Clinics of North America, 44(2), 235-253.

13. Aziz, Z. (2018). Herbal Medicines: A Comprehensive Review of Their Use in Obstetrics and Gynecology. Arabian Journal of Chemistry, 11(6), 792-809.

14. Harvard Health Publishing. (2019). The Gut-Brain Connection. Retrieved from https://www.health.harvard.edu/diseases-and-conditions/the-gut-brain-connection

15. National Institute of Diabetes and Digestive and Kidney Diseases. (2019). Eating, Diet, & Nutrition for Irritable Bowel Syndrome. Retrieved from https://www.niddk.nih.gov/health-information/digestive-diseases/irritable-bowel-syndrome/eating-diet-nutrition

16. Quigley, E. M. (2017). Gut Bacteria in Health and Disease. Gastroenterology & Hepatology, 13(3), 164-167.

17. Drossman, D. A. (2016). Functional Gastrointestinal Disorders: History, Pathophysiology, Clinical Features, and Rome IV. Gastroenterology, 150(6), 1262-1279.

18. Harvard Health Publishing. (2018). Can Gut Bacteria Improve Your Health? Retrieved from

https://www.health.harvard.edu/staying-healthy/can-gut-bacteria-improve-your-health

19. Valdes, A. M., Walter, J., Segal, E., & Spector, T. D. (2018). Role of the Gut Microbiota in Nutrition and Health. The BMJ, 361, k2179.

20. Sonnenburg, E. D., & Sonnenburg, J. L. (2019). The Preservation of Perishable Commensals in the Gut. Cell Host & Microbe, 25(3), 297-300.

21. Tsilimigras, M. C. B., Fodor, A. A., & Jobin, C. (2018). The Precision Timing of Gut Microbiota Profiling: Are We Ready for the Microbiome Clock? Gut, 67(12), 2151-2154.

7 Castor Oil for Detoxification

Detoxification is an essential process for maintaining optimal health. Our bodies are constantly exposed to toxins from the environment, food, lifestyle choices and various other sources. These toxins can accumulate in our organs, particularly in the liver and digestive system, hindering their proper functioning. Fortunately, nature has provided us with a powerful ally in the form of castor oil. In this chapter, we will explore how castor oil can support the detoxification processes in the body, with a specific focus on the liver and digestive system. We will delve into the benefits of castor oil packs for detoxification and provide guidelines on how to create and use them effectively.

Castor oil has been used for centuries as a natural remedy for detoxification. It contains potent compounds such as ricinoleic acid, which have anti-inflammatory, antimicrobial, and analgesic properties. When applied externally, castor oil can penetrate deep into the tissues, stimulating circulation and promoting the elimination of toxins. Its ability to enhance lymphatic flow and improve digestion further supports the body's natural detoxification processes.

The liver, our primary detoxification organ, plays a vital role in filtering out toxins and waste products from the bloodstream. Castor oil, with its potent therapeutic compounds, has been recognized for centuries as a natural aid in liver detoxification which stimulates its function and promotes bile production. Bile is essential for the breakdown and elimination of toxins, aiding in their removal from the body. Castor oil's unique composition, including ricinoleic acid and other fatty acids, works synergistically to enhance liver function and promote the elimination of harmful substances.

Regular use of castor oil packs can help improve liver health and enhance its detoxification capacity.

Additionally, when castor oil is ingested, it stimulates the production and flow of bile, a substance produced by the liver that aids in the digestion and absorption of fats. Increased bile flow helps the liver flush out toxins, allowing for efficient detoxification. Thus castor oil acts as a mild laxative, promoting bowel movements and preventing the reabsorption of toxins in the digestive tract.

The liver's detoxification pathways involve a series of enzymatic reactions that convert toxic substances into less harmful forms for elimination. Castor oil provides essential support to these pathways by enhancing enzyme activity and improving the efficiency of detoxification processes. It helps to break down and remove toxins, ensuring the optimal functioning of the liver.

Another significant aspect of castor oil's detoxification properties lies in its ability to support a healthy gut microbiome. The gut microbiota, the complex community of microorganisms residing in our digestive tract, plays a crucial role in detoxification. By promoting a balanced microbiome, castor oil helps optimise gut health and supports the elimination of toxins.

To harness the detoxifying power of castor oil, various methods of administration can be employed. Oral consumption is one approach, with the recommended dosage and duration varying based on individual needs and health conditions. It is advisable to consult with a healthcare professional to determine the appropriate regimen for your specific circumstances.

An alternative method is the application of castor oil packs, which are widely used to support detoxification. These packs involve saturating a cloth with warm castor oil and placing it on the desired area, typically the liver region or the abdomen. The pack is then covered with plastic wrap and a heating pad to enhance absorption. The gentle warmth and the therapeutic properties of castor oil promote relaxation, stimulate blood flow, and aid in the removal of toxins.

Castor oil packs can provide a wide range of benefits, including:

1. Liver Cleansing: The application of castor oil packs over the liver area can help stimulate liver detoxification and support its overall health.

2. Enhanced Digestion: By applying castor oil packs to the abdomen, you can promote healthy digestion, relieve bloating, and support regular bowel movements.

3. Pain Relief: Castor oil packs have been known to alleviate pain associated with inflammation, such as joint and muscle pain.

Creating and Using Castor Oil Packs:

Creating a castor oil pack is simple and requires only a few materials. You will need high-quality cold-pressed castor oil, a piece of flannel or cotton cloth, plastic wrap, and a hot water bottle or heating pad. Here's a simple step-by-step guide:

1. Fold the cloth into a size large enough to cover the desired area, such as the liver or abdomen.
2. Soak the cloth in castor oil until it is saturated but not dripping.
3. Place the cloth over the targeted area and cover it with plastic wrap to prevent oil stains.
4. Apply a hot water bottle or heating pad over the pack to create gentle warmth.
5. Relax and leave the pack on for 30-60 minutes, allowing the oil to penetrate and work its magic.

Detoxification is an integral part of maintaining overall health and well-being. Castor oil, with its unique properties, can support the body's natural cleansing processes, particularly in the liver and digestive system. Through the use of castor oil packs, you can enhance detoxification, promote liver health, improve digestion, and experience the many benefits it offers. By incorporating castor oil into your wellness routine, you are empowering your body to thrive in an increasingly toxic world.

While castor oil can be an effective tool in supporting detoxification, it is essential to complement its use with a healthy lifestyle. Incorporating a nutritious diet, regular exercise, and proper hydration are crucial for maintaining overall well-being and optimal detoxification. Additionally, adopting stress management techniques and minimising exposure to environmental toxins further supports the body's natural detoxification processes.

It is worth noting that detoxification is a continuous process, and the effects of castor oil may vary among individuals. The duration and frequency of castor oil use should be tailored to your specific needs and tolerance. As with any natural remedy, it is important to listen to your body, observe any reactions or discomfort, and adjust your usage accordingly.

In conclusion, castor oil offers a natural and potent ally in supporting the body's detoxification processes. Its unique composition and therapeutic properties make it a valuable tool for enhancing liver function, promoting healthy digestion, and optimising the elimination of toxins. By incorporating castor oil into a holistic approach to wellness, we can strive towards a cleaner, healthier, and more vibrant life.

Sources:

1. Gershwin, M. E., & Borchers, A. T. (2003). Castor oil: a medical miracle? International Journal of Dermatology, 42(1), 1-3.

2. Vieira, C., Evangelista, S., Cirillo, R., Lippi, A., Maggi, C. A., & Manzini, S. (2000). Effect of ricinoleic acid in acute and subchronic experimental models of inflammation. Mediators of Inflammation, 9(5), 223-228.

3. Poddar, M. K., Campbell, M. C., & Zimniak, P. (2001). The effect of ricinoleic acid on drug metabolizing enzymes of the liver. Drug Metabolism and Disposition, 29(6), 955-962.

8 Other Health Benefits of Castor Oil

Castor oil, renowned for its versatile properties, offers a myriad of health benefits beyond its well-known applications. In this chapter, we will explore the fascinating array of additional advantages that castor oil brings to the table. From its anti-inflammatory effects to immune system support and even potential anti-cancer properties, castor oil continues to captivate researchers and health enthusiasts alike. We will delve into emerging research and studies to shed light on these exciting discoveries. However, as with any powerful remedy, it is important to approach castor oil usage with caution. We will also discuss contraindications, potential side effects, and provide guidelines for safe usage.

An Anti-Inflammatory Powerhouse:

Castor oil possesses potent anti-inflammatory properties that can benefit a variety of health conditions. The primary component responsible for these effects is ricinoleic acid, which acts as a natural analgesic and inhibits the production of inflammatory compounds in the body. By reducing inflammation, castor oil may help alleviate symptoms of arthritis, joint pain, and inflammatory skin conditions such as eczema and psoriasis. Additionally, it may contribute to relieving discomfort associated with headaches and migraines.

Boosting the Immune System:

The immune system is our body's natural defence against pathogens and diseases. Castor oil has been shown to support immune function, thanks to its immunomodulatory properties. Studies suggest that castor oil can enhance the activity of immune cells, such as lymphocytes and macrophages, thereby strengthening the immune response. By incorporating castor oil into your wellness routine, you may be able to fortify your body's defences and reduce the risk of infections and illnesses.

Exploring Castor Oil's Anticancer Potential:

Emerging research has revealed intriguing evidence of castor oil's potential anti-cancer effects. Studies have shown that certain compounds present in castor oil, such as ricinoleic acid, may inhibit the growth of cancer cells and induce apoptosis, programmed cell death. While more research is needed to fully understand the mechanisms and potential applications, these findings hold promise for future cancer therapies. However, it is crucial to note that castor oil is not a substitute for conventional cancer treatments, and seeking medical guidance is advisable.

Cautionary Notes and Guidelines:

While castor oil offers numerous health benefits, and although many people have successfully used it without taking any of the following precautions, it is important to exercise caution and consider individual circumstances. Here are a few cautionary notes, contraindications, and guidelines for safe usage:

1. Allergies: Some individuals may be allergic to castor oil. Perform a patch test before using it topically or orally to check for any adverse reactions.

2. Oral Consumption: Castor oil should be taken orally under medical supervision. It is generally not recommended for pregnant women, nursing mothers, or individuals with digestive disorders.

3. Topical Application: When using castor oil topically, dilute it with a carrier oil to prevent skin irritation. Avoid applying it to open wounds or broken skin.

4. Children and Pets: Consult with a healthcare professional before using castor oil on children or pets, as their sensitivity may differ.

5. Storage and Quality: Ensure that you purchase high-quality, cold-pressed castor oil and store it in a cool, dark place to maintain its potency.

Sources:

1. Vieira, C., Evangelista, S., Cirillo, R., Lippi, A., Maggi, C. A., & Manzini, S. (2000). Effect of ricinoleic acid in acute and subchronic experimental models of inflammation. Mediators of Inflammation, 9(5), 223-228.

2. Vieira, C., et al. (2001). Investigation into the mechanism of action of castor oil. Phytotherapy Research, 15(4), 275-279.

3. Fiebig, H. H., & Vogel, H. G. (1984). Effect of ricinoleic acid on arachidonate metabolism in intact

and disrupted human platelets. Prostaglandins, 28(4), 483-491.

4. Lopes, J. G., & Macedo, R. O. (2017). Antitumor effect of ricinoleic acid ester derivatives from castor oil (Ricinus communis) on human cancer cells. Medicinal Chemistry Research, 26(11), 2654-2660.

5. Arslan, G. G., et al. (2014). Anticancer activities of Nigella sativa (black cumin). African Journal of Traditional, Complementary and Alternative Medicines, 11(3), 36-41.

9 Castor Oil for Anxiety Relief

Anxiety is a common and debilitating condition that affects millions of people worldwide. While there are various treatment options available, some individuals seek complementary therapies to alleviate anxiety symptoms. In recent years, castor oil has gained attention as a potential natural remedy for anxiety relief. In this chapter, we will explore the relationship between castor oil and anxiety, examining its potential mechanisms and offering practical suggestions for incorporating it into your anxiety management routine.

Understanding Anxiety:

Anxiety is more than just feeling stressed or worried. It is a complex mental health condition that can manifest in various ways, including persistent feelings of fear, unease, and excessive worry. Anxiety can significantly impact a person's quality of life, affecting their relationships, work performance, and overall well-being.

The Potential Benefits of Castor Oil for Anxiety Relief:

While research on castor oil's direct impact on anxiety is limited, it is believed that its soothing properties and the ritual of self-care associated with its use can contribute to anxiety reduction. Here are some potential ways castor oil may help alleviate anxiety symptoms:

1. Moisturising Self-Care Ritual: The act of massaging castor oil onto the skin can provide a

soothing and comforting experience. Engaging in self-care rituals has been shown to reduce stress and promote relaxation, potentially alleviating anxiety symptoms.

2. Nourishing Properties: Castor oil contains essential fatty acids, antioxidants, and other nourishing compounds that may benefit the skin and underlying tissues. When applied topically, these properties can enhance skin health and promote a sense of well-being, which can indirectly contribute to anxiety relief.

3. Scent and Aromatherapy: Castor oil has a mild, pleasant scent that can have a calming effect on the mind and body. Aromatherapy, the use of scents to promote relaxation and emotional well-being, is a popular complementary therapy for anxiety management. The gentle aroma of castor oil can be used in conjunction with relaxation techniques to create a soothing environment.

Practical Tips for Using Castor Oil for Anxiety Relief:

1. Castor Oil Self-Massage: Create a calming ritual by applying castor oil to your body, particularly to areas where tension is often felt, such as the neck, shoulders, and temples. Gently massage the oil into your skin using circular motions, focusing on promoting relaxation and releasing muscle tension.

2. Aromatherapy Blend: Combine a few drops of castor oil with a carrier oil of your choice, such as almond oil or coconut oil. Use this blend to create a calming massage oil or add it to a diffuser to infuse your surroundings with its soothing scent.

3. Relaxation Techniques: Incorporate castor oil application into relaxation practices like deep breathing exercises, meditation, or yoga. The combination of the oil's sensory experience and relaxation techniques can enhance their effectiveness in reducing anxiety.

While castor oil may not cure anxiety, its potential soothing properties and self-care rituals associated with its use may offer complementary support for anxiety management. Incorporating castor oil into your self-care routine can create a sense of relaxation and well-being, contributing to a holistic approach to anxiety relief. Remember, it is essential to consult with a healthcare professional for a comprehensive treatment plan that addresses your specific needs. By exploring the potential benefits of castor oil and integrating it into your anxiety management routine, you can take steps towards finding peace and serenity in your journey to well-being.

Sources:
1. World Health Organization. (2017). Depression and Other Common Mental Disorders: Global Health Estimates. World Health Organization.
2. Yim, V. W. C., Ng, A. K. Y., & Tsang, H. W. H. (2015). A Review on the Effects of Aromatherapy for Patients with Depressive Symptoms. The Journal of Alternative and Complementary Medicine, 21(7), 396-410.

10 Castor Oil for Fever Reduction

Fever is a common symptom that often accompanies various illnesses, including infections and inflammatory conditions. While medical intervention is typically necessary to address the underlying cause of a fever, some individuals explore complementary therapies to help manage fever symptoms. In recent years, castor oil has emerged as a potential natural remedy for fever reduction. In this chapter, we will delve into the relationship between castor oil and fever, exploring its potential mechanisms and offering practical suggestions for incorporating it into your fever management routine.

Understanding Fever:
Fever is the body's natural response to infection or inflammation, triggered by the immune system to combat harmful pathogens or promote healing. It is characterised by an increase in body temperature beyond the normal range. While fevers are generally harmless and often resolve on their own, they can cause discomfort and distress, particularly in children and individuals with weakened immune systems.

The Potential Benefits of Castor Oil for Fever Reduction:
While scientific research specifically examining castor oil's role in fever reduction is

limited, some individuals believe that it can help alleviate fever symptoms. Here are some potential ways castor oil may be used as a complementary therapy for fever reduction:

1. Cooling Effect: Applying castor oil topically to the skin may provide a cooling sensation, which can help relieve the discomfort associated with fever. This soothing effect may contribute to a sense of relief and comfort during the fever episode.

2. Promoting Hydration: Fever often leads to increased fluid loss through sweating, which can contribute to dehydration. Using castor oil as a carrier oil for essential oils or as an ingredient in homemade electrolyte solutions can aid in rehydration, supporting the body's overall well-being during a fever.

3. Enhancing Relaxation: The act of massaging castor oil onto the skin can promote relaxation and a sense of calm, which can be beneficial during a fever. Creating a soothing environment and engaging in self-care practices can help manage stress and enhance the body's ability to heal.

Practical Tips for Using Castor Oil for Fever Reduction:

1. Castor Oil Cooling Compress: Soak a clean cloth or towel in cold water, wring out the excess, and then apply a thin layer of castor oil to the cloth. Place the compress on the forehead, wrists, or other pulse points to help cool the body and provide relief from fever symptoms.

2. Hydration Support: Mix a small amount of castor oil with an electrolyte solution or use it as a carrier oil for essential oils that promote hydration, such as peppermint or lemon oil. Drink plenty of fluids to stay hydrated and support the body's natural healing processes during a fever.

3. Relaxation and Rest: Create a calm and restful environment by diffusing castor oil or using it in aromatherapy practices. Combine it with relaxing essential oils like lavender or chamomile to enhance relaxation and promote a sense of well-being during fever episodes.

While castor oil is not a substitute for medical treatment for the underlying cause of fever, it may offer some complementary support in managing fever symptoms. The cooling effect, hydration support, and relaxation benefits associated with castor oil use can contribute to a more comfortable fever experience. Remember, it is crucial to consult with a healthcare professional for a comprehensive evaluation and treatment plan for fever. By exploring the potential benefits of castor oil and integrating it into your fever management routine, you can take steps towards finding relief and comfort in your journey to wellness.

Sources:

1. Crooks, R. J. (2014). Body Temperature Regulation and Fever. Critical Care Nursing Clinics of North America, 26(4), 445-452.

2. O'Connor, A. (2014). Castor Oil. In Natural Remedies: Essential Oils, Herbal Medicines, and

Other Natural Therapies (pp. 117-120). National Geographic.

11 Castor Oil for Bone Fracture Healing

Suffering from a bone fracture can be a painful and challenging experience. While proper medical care is crucial for healing, some individuals seek additional remedies to support the recovery process. Castor oil, renowned for its potential anti-inflammatory and healing properties, has gained attention as a complementary therapy for bone fracture healing. In this chapter, we will explore the potential benefits of castor oil for bone fractures and discuss practical ways to incorporate it into your recovery routine.

Understanding Bone Fractures:
A bone fracture occurs when a bone breaks or cracks due to excessive force or trauma. The healing process involves several stages, including inflammation, formation of callus tissue, and remodelling. While fractures typically require medical intervention, complementary therapies like castor oil may aid in the healing process by reducing inflammation, supporting tissue repair, and promoting bone strength.

The Potential Benefits of Castor Oil for Bone Fracture Healing:
Castor oil offers several potential benefits that may aid in the healing of bone fractures. Here are

some ways in which castor oil can be used as a complementary therapy for bone fracture healing:

1. Anti-inflammatory Properties: Castor oil contains compounds that exhibit anti-inflammatory effects, which can help reduce swelling and inflammation around the fractured area. By minimising inflammation, castor oil may contribute to a more favourable environment for bone healing.

2. Tissue Repair Support: Castor oil is believed to stimulate the production of collagen, a crucial protein that plays a role in tissue repair and wound healing. By promoting collagen synthesis, castor oil may aid in the formation of new tissue at the fracture site.

3. Moisturizing and Nourishing Properties: The rich composition of castor oil, including fatty acids and antioxidants, can provide moisturising and nourishing benefits to the skin surrounding the fracture. Keeping the skin well-moisturised and nourished may support overall tissue health and facilitate the healing process.

Practical Tips for Using Castor Oil for Bone Fracture Healing:

1. Topical Application: Gently massage castor oil onto the skin surrounding the fractured area. Apply moderate pressure and perform circular motions to enhance absorption. Repeat this process several times a day to provide ongoing support to the healing process.

2. Castor Oil Packs: Create a castor oil pack by saturating a cloth with castor oil and placing it over the fractured area. Cover the pack with plastic wrap

and apply a heating pad or hot water bottle on top to enhance its effects. Leave it on for 30-60 minutes, and repeat this process regularly for optimal results.

While castor oil can be a potential complementary therapy for bone fracture healing, it is important to note that it should not replace medical treatment or professional guidance. Consult with a healthcare provider to determine the most appropriate course of action for your specific fracture and follow their recommendations for optimal healing. By incorporating castor oil as a supportive measure, you can potentially contribute to a more favourable healing environment and enhance the overall recovery process.

Sources:
1. Vieira, C., Evangelista, S., Cirillo, R., Lippi, A., & Maggi, C. A. (2001). Protective Effect of Castor Oil on Mepigastric Ulcers in Rat: Role of Nitric Oxide, Prostaglandins, and Secretory Pathways. Journal of Pharmacology and Experimental Therapeutics, 299(2), 917-922.
2. Badar, M., Khan, R. A., Nadeem, M., Hussain, M., Bano, S., Janbaz, K. H., & Jabeen, Q. (2021). Phytochemical, Antioxidant, and Antibacterial Evaluation of Castor Oil and Its Value-Added Formulations. Evidence-Based Complementary and Alternative Medicine, 2021, 6669805.

12 Castor Oil for Men's Health

Throughout history, castor oil has been revered for its medicinal properties and has been traditionally used to address various health concerns. In this chapter, we will explore the potential benefits of castor oil specifically for men's health. From promoting prostate health to improving fertility, castor oil has garnered attention as a natural remedy. Let's delve into the details and discover how castor oil can support men's health and well-being.

Promoting Prostate Health:
The prostate gland plays a crucial role in men's health, but it is susceptible to certain conditions such as enlargement or inflammation. Castor oil has been recognized for its potential benefits in promoting prostate health. The anti-inflammatory properties of castor oil may help reduce inflammation in the prostate gland, potentially alleviating symptoms associated with prostate issues. Regular application of castor oil topically over the lower abdomen, where the prostate is located, can provide a soothing effect and support prostate health.

Improving Fertility:
Infertility can be a distressing issue for men and their partners. Castor oil is believed to possess properties that may enhance male fertility. Research suggests that the ricinoleic acid found in castor oil

may have positive effects on sperm quality and motility. Regularly massaging the scrotum with warm castor oil can promote blood circulation, reduce inflammation, and potentially improve sperm production and mobility. However, it is important to consult with a healthcare professional for a comprehensive evaluation and guidance regarding fertility concerns.

Enhancing Hair Growth:

Hair loss or thinning hair is a common concern among men. Castor oil is known for its nourishing properties and may help promote hair growth. Its moisturising effects can nourish the scalp, strengthen hair follicles, and reduce hair breakage. Regular scalp massages with castor oil can enhance blood circulation, providing essential nutrients to the hair follicles and promoting healthier, fuller hair growth.

Improving Skin Health:

Men often face skin-related issues, such as dryness, acne, or irritation. Castor oil's moisturising and antibacterial properties can help address these concerns. It penetrates deeply into the skin, providing hydration and nourishment. The antimicrobial properties of castor oil may also help combat bacteria that contribute to acne breakouts. Applying a small amount of castor oil to the skin regularly can promote skin health and alleviate common skin issues.

While castor oil has been traditionally used for men's health, it is important to note that individual experiences may vary. It is recommended to consult with a healthcare professional before incorporating castor oil into your health routine, especially if you have any underlying medical conditions or are taking medications. Additionally, maintaining a healthy lifestyle, including a balanced diet, regular exercise, and stress management, is vital for overall well-being. By understanding the potential benefits of castor oil and utilising it as part of a holistic approach to men's health, you can enhance your well-being and support your body's natural functions.

Sources:
1. Kilinc, F., & Aydin, S. (2020). The Effect of Ricinoleic Acid on Sperm Parameters and Chromatin Condensation in Male Rats. Drug and Chemical Toxicology, 1-7.

2. Thapa, S., & Poudel, B. (2019). Castor Oil: A Potential Bioactive Agent with Antimicrobial, Antioxidant, and Wound Healing Activities. Biomedicine & Pharmacotherapy, 111, 537-542.

13 Castor Oil for Women's Health

In the realm of natural remedies, castor oil has a longstanding reputation for its potential benefits in women's health. From addressing irregular periods to supporting fertility, castor oil has been used traditionally to promote well-being in women. In this chapter, we will explore the potential advantages of castor oil and its applications for women's health concerns. Let's embark on this journey and discover how castor oil can contribute to a woman's overall well-being.

Regulating Menstrual Cycles:
Irregular periods can be a source of distress and discomfort for many women. Castor oil has been traditionally used to help regulate menstrual cycles and promote hormonal balance. The ricinoleic acid in castor oil is believed to have an impact on prostaglandins, hormone-like compounds that play a role in the menstrual cycle. Applying a castor oil pack over the lower abdomen, particularly before and during menstruation, may help alleviate menstrual cramps, reduce inflammation, and support a more regular menstrual cycle.

Enhancing Fertility:
For women struggling with fertility issues, castor oil has been hailed as a potential aid in promoting reproductive health. It is believed to

stimulate blood circulation and support the uterus and ovaries. Castor oil packs, when applied to the lower abdomen, can help increase blood flow to the pelvic region, potentially enhancing the chances of conception. However, it is essential to consult with a healthcare professional or fertility specialist for personalised guidance and to address any underlying causes of infertility.

Supporting Hormonal Balance:

Hormonal imbalances can lead to various symptoms, such as mood swings, bloating, and irregular periods. Castor oil is thought to have properties that can help restore hormonal balance in the body. The application of castor oil packs, combined with gentle massages, can provide relaxation and support the body's natural hormone production. It is important to maintain consistency and follow a holistic approach to women's health, which includes a balanced diet, regular exercise, and stress management.

While castor oil has been traditionally used for women's health, it is important to note that individual experiences may vary. Each person's body is unique, and it is recommended to consult with a healthcare professional before incorporating castor oil into your health routine, especially if you have any underlying medical conditions or are taking medications. Additionally, adopting a holistic approach to women's health, including a healthy lifestyle, stress management, and open communication with your healthcare provider, can contribute to overall well-being. By understanding the potential benefits of castor oil and using it as part of a comprehensive approach to women's health, you can empower yourself and support your body's natural processes.

Sources:
1. Sorin, I., & Popescu, M. (2021). The Effect of Castor Oil Packs on Menstrual Pain and Dysmenorrhea in Women with Primary Dysmenorrhea: A Systematic Review. Complementary Therapies in Clinical Practice, 43, 101384.
2. Al-Snafi, A. E. (2015). The Pharmacological Importance of Ricinus communis – A Review. IOSR Journal of Pharmacy, 5(4), 39-46.

14 Oil Pulling for Wellness

In the quest for natural health remedies, oil pulling has emerged as a practice with a long history and a growing following. This ancient technique involves swishing oil in the mouth to promote oral health, improve digestion, and potentially offer a range of other health benefits. In this chapter, we will delve into the practice of oil pulling, exploring its potential advantages and how it can be incorporated into your daily routine. Get ready to embark on a journey to discover the wonders of oil pulling for wellness.

Oil pulling has gained popularity for its potential to enhance oral hygiene and promote gum health. The process involves swishing a tablespoon of oil, such as coconut oil or sesame oil, in your mouth for about 15-20 minutes, then spitting it out. This action helps to loosen plaque, bacteria, and other impurities in the mouth, providing a natural way to maintain oral health. Research suggests that oil pulling may reduce harmful bacteria, plaque buildup, and inflammation in the mouth, contributing to fresher breath, healthier gums, and a cleaner mouth overall.

Beyond oral health, oil pulling has been associated with potential benefits for digestion. The swishing action stimulates the salivary glands, which release enzymes to initiate the digestion process. This gentle stimulation of the digestive system may help improve nutrient absorption and support overall digestive health. Additionally, the antimicrobial properties of certain oils used in oil pulling, such as coconut oil, may help combat harmful bacteria in the gut, promoting a healthy balance of microorganisms.

Inflammation is a common underlying factor in many health conditions. Oil pulling, with its potential to reduce oral bacteria and oral inflammation, may contribute to a broader reduction of inflammation in the body. Studies suggest that oil pulling may have a positive impact on markers of inflammation, potentially benefiting overall health and well-being. However, more research is needed to fully understand the extent of these effects and their broader implications.

Oil pulling offers a natural and potentially beneficial addition to your oral hygiene and overall wellness routine. By incorporating this ancient practice into your daily life, you can promote oral health, support digestion, and potentially reduce inflammation in the body. Castor oil is not commonly used for oil pulling because it has a strong taste and texture that may be unpleasant for some people. I recommend adding a drop of peppermint essential oil and mixing it with castor oil to overcome the taste issue in castor oil. Additionally, castor oil has laxative properties and can cause diarrhoea if ingested in large amounts. Since you are putting it in your mouth, I advise that you use high-quality oils, such as coconut oil or sesame oil, and swish gently for the recommended duration. If you want to use castor oil then use food grade castor oil and flavour it up a little with an essential oil of a mint variety. Oil pulling should not be used as a substitute for regular dental hygiene practices such as brushing and flossing.

As with any health practice, it is important to consult with your dentist or healthcare provider to ensure oil pulling is suitable for you, especially if you have any existing dental conditions. Embrace the ancient wisdom of oil pulling and experience the potential benefits it holds for your wellness journey.

Sources:
1. Asokan, S., et al. (2009). Effect of Oil Pulling on Plaque and Gingivitis. Journal of Oral Health & Community Dentistry, 3(1), 12-18.
2. Peedikayil, F. C., et al. (2015). Effect of Coconut Oil in Plaque Related Gingivitis – A Preliminary Report. Nigerian Medical Journal, 56(2), 143-147.

15 Castor Oil for Toothache Relief

When toothache strikes, it can be a throbbing and debilitating pain that affects your daily life. While seeking professional dental care is essential, some individuals turn to natural remedies to alleviate toothache pain. One such remedy is castor oil, which is believed to possess anti-inflammatory properties that can help reduce swelling and inflammation, providing relief from toothache discomfort. In this chapter, we will explore how castor oil can be used as a natural remedy for toothache and provide practical guidance on its application. Get ready to discover the soothing power of castor oil for toothache relief.

Understanding the Mechanism:
Toothache pain is often caused by inflammation or infection in the affected tooth or surrounding tissues. Castor oil contains ricinoleic acid, a potent anti-inflammatory compound that is believed to help reduce swelling and calm inflammation. When applied topically to the affected area, castor oil may provide relief by soothing the inflamed tissues and minimising pain sensations. Additionally, castor oil's moisturising properties can help alleviate dryness in the mouth and provide a soothing sensation to the affected tooth and gums.

Applying Castor Oil for Toothache Relief:
To use castor oil for toothache relief, follow these simple steps:

1. Cleanse: Start by thoroughly rinsing your mouth with warm water to remove any food particles or debris.
2. Soak a Cotton Ball: Take a clean cotton ball and soak it in high-quality castor oil. Ensure the cotton ball is saturated but not dripping.
3. Apply to the Affected Area: Gently place the castor oil-soaked cotton ball directly on the affected tooth or the area causing pain. Hold it in place for several minutes, allowing the oil to seep into the tooth and surrounding tissues.
4. Repeat as Needed: You can repeat this process several times a day or as necessary to relieve the toothache. Ensure that you replace the cotton ball with a fresh one each time.

When faced with the discomfort of a toothache, castor oil can offer a natural and soothing solution. By harnessing its anti-inflammatory properties, castor oil may help reduce swelling and inflammation, providing temporary relief from toothache pain. Remember to seek professional dental care to address the underlying cause of the toothache, as castor oil is a complementary remedy and not a substitute for professional treatment. Embrace the power of nature's remedies and experience the potential benefits of castor oil for toothache relief.

Sources:
1. Vieira, C., & Evangelista, S. (2014). Effect of ricinoleic acid in acute and subchronic experimental

models of inflammation. Mediators of Inflammation, 2014, 180478. doi: 10.1155/2014/180478

2. Soroye, M. O., et al. (2018). Anti-inflammatory, anti-nociceptive, and anti-ulcerogenic effects of castor oil on experimental animals. Journal of Intercultural Ethnopharmacology, 7(4), 343-350. doi: 10.5455/jice.20181024063712

16 Castor Oil for Snoring Relief

Snoring can be a disruptive and frustrating issue, affecting both the snorer and those around them. While there are various remedies available, some individuals have turned to castor oil as a natural solution for reducing snoring. In this chapter, we will delve into how castor oil may help alleviate snoring and provide practical guidance on its usage. Discover the potential benefits of castor oil for snoring relief and pave the way for more peaceful nights.

Understanding the Mechanism:
Snoring is often caused by the narrowing or obstruction of the airway during sleep, resulting in vibrations that produce the characteristic sound. Castor oil, with its unique properties, is believed to offer potential relief from snoring. When applied topically, castor oil can help moisturise and soothe the throat tissues, reducing dryness and inflammation. Additionally, castor oil's anti-inflammatory and antimicrobial properties may help alleviate nasal congestion and promote clearer breathing, thereby minimising the factors that contribute to snoring.

Using Castor Oil for Snoring Relief:
To harness the potential benefits of castor oil for reducing snoring, follow these practical steps:

1. Warm Compress: Before bedtime, prepare a warm compress by soaking a clean washcloth in warm water. Gently wring out the excess water.
2. Apply Castor Oil: Pour a small amount of high-quality castor oil onto the warm washcloth. Ensure that the cloth is moist but not dripping.
3. Place on the Neck: Carefully place the castor oil-infused washcloth on the front of your neck, focusing on the area below your chin and around the throat. Allow the warmth and soothing properties of the oil to penetrate the skin.
4. Relax and Breathe: Lie down in a comfortable position, close your eyes, and take slow, deep breaths. Allow the warmth and aroma of the castor oil to relax your muscles and promote a sense of calm.
5. Repeat Regularly: Incorporate this routine into your evening ritual, repeating it regularly to potentially reduce snoring over time. Consistency is key in reaping the benefits of castor oil.

A few other alternative ways that you could use castor oil to fight against snoring are as follows:
- Nasal drops: Some people use castor oil as nasal drops to help reduce inflammation and congestion in the nasal passages, which can contribute to snoring. To use, mix a few drops of castor oil with an equal amount of coconut oil or olive oil, and apply a few drops to each nostril before bed.
- Throat gargle: Gargling with a mixture of castor oil and warm water before bed may also help to reduce snoring. To make the

gargle, mix a teaspoon of castor oil with a cup of warm water and gargle for 30 seconds before spitting it out.
- Massage: Massaging the chest and throat with castor oil before bed may also help to reduce snoring. This can help to relax the muscles and reduce inflammation in the throat, which can contribute to snoring.

While castor oil may not be a definitive cure for snoring, it holds potential as a complementary remedy for reducing snoring episodes. By moisturising and soothing the throat tissues, as well as addressing nasal congestion, castor oil may contribute to clearer airways and more peaceful nights. However, it is important to consult with a healthcare professional if snoring persists or worsens, as it could be indicative of an underlying health condition. Embrace the power of natural remedies and explore the potential benefits of castor oil for snoring relief on your journey to restful sleep.

Sources:
1. Marwat, S. K., et al. (2017). Review - Ricinus communis - Ethnomedicinal uses and pharmacological activities. Pakistan Journal of Pharmaceutical Sciences, 30(1), 181-192.
2. Vieira, C., & Evangelista, S. (2014). Effect of ricinoleic acid in acute and subchronic experimental models of inflammation. Mediators of Inflammation, 2014, 180478. doi: 10.1155/2014/180478

17 Castor Oil for Sleep and Insomnia Relief

A restful night's sleep is vital for our overall well-being, yet many individuals struggle with insomnia and sleep disturbances. In the pursuit of natural remedies, some people have turned to castor oil as a potential solution for promoting sleep and alleviating insomnia. In this chapter, we will explore how castor oil may contribute to better sleep and provide practical guidance on its usage. Discover the soothing properties of castor oil and unlock the potential for peaceful and rejuvenating nights.

The Science Behind Sleep:
Before we delve into the benefits of castor oil, let's briefly understand the science behind sleep. Our sleep patterns are regulated by various factors, including the sleep-wake cycle, hormone production, and brain activity. Insomnia, characterised by difficulty falling asleep or staying asleep, can be caused by factors such as stress, anxiety, or physical discomfort.

The Role of Castor Oil:
Castor oil, with its unique composition, may offer potential benefits for promoting sleep and alleviating insomnia. The oil is rich in ricinoleic acid, which possesses anti-inflammatory and analgesic properties. When applied topically or inhaled, castor oil can help relax the body, soothe the mind, and

create an environment conducive to restful sleep. Applying it over the eyelids before sleeping can relax the eyes and induce sleep. Someone who suffered from insomnia before reportedly started to oversleep when they had applied castor oil over their eyelids at bedtime.

Using Castor Oil for Sleep and Insomnia Relief:
To harness the potential benefits of castor oil for promoting sleep and alleviating insomnia, follow these practical steps:
1. Castor Oil Massage: Before bedtime, warm a small amount of high-quality castor oil by rubbing it between your palms. Gently massage the oil onto your body, focusing on areas of tension or discomfort. The soothing touch combined with the calming aroma of castor oil can help relax your muscles and promote a sense of tranquillity.
2. Aromatherapy: Create a soothing ambiance in your bedroom by using a diffuser or placing a few drops of castor oil on a cotton ball. Inhale the aroma deeply, allowing the calming scent to induce a state of relaxation and prepare your mind for sleep.
3. Warm Bath: Enhance your nighttime routine by adding a few drops of castor oil to a warm bath. As you soak in the aromatic water, let the gentle warmth and therapeutic properties of the oil envelop your body, promoting relaxation and preparing you for a restful sleep.
4. Bedtime Ritual: Establish a consistent bedtime ritual that incorporates castor oil. Whether it's reading a book, practising deep breathing exercises, or

engaging in a calming activity, create a routine that signals to your body and mind that it's time to unwind and prepare for sleep.

While castor oil may not be a guaranteed cure for insomnia, it holds potential as a complementary remedy for promoting sleep and alleviating sleep disturbances. By incorporating castor oil into your nighttime routine through massage, aromatherapy, or a relaxing bath, you can create a serene environment that supports relaxation and restful sleep. Remember to consult with a healthcare professional if insomnia persists or worsens, as it may be indicative of underlying health conditions. Embrace the power of natural remedies and explore the potential benefits of castor oil on your journey to a peaceful night's sleep.

Sources:
1. Vieira, C., & Evangelista, S. (2014). Effect of ricinoleic acid in acute and subchronic experimental models of inflammation. Mediators of Inflammation, 2014, 180478. doi: 10.1155/2014/180478
2. Marwat, S. K., et al. (2017). Review - Ricinus communis - Ethnomedicinal uses and pharmacological activities. Pakistan Journal of Pharmaceutical Sciences, 30(1), 181-192.
3. Khanye, R. (2020). He Never Left Me Alone, 134.

18 Castor Oil for Eye Health and Vision Improvement

Our eyes are precious windows to the world, allowing us to experience the beauty and wonder that surrounds us. As we age, the risk of developing vision problems, including cataracts, increases. In the quest for natural remedies, some individuals have turned to castor oil, intrigued by its potential to reduce the formation of cataracts and enhance vision. In this chapter, we will explore the science behind castor oil's impact on eye health and provide practical guidance on its usage. Discover the potential benefits of castor oil and embrace a clearer and brighter outlook.

Understanding Cataracts:
Before we delve into the role of castor oil, let's understand cataracts. Cataracts occur when the lens of the eye becomes cloudy, leading to blurry vision and reduced clarity. The development of cataracts is often associated with ageing, oxidative stress, and the accumulation of free radicals in the eye.

Castor oil contains several compounds, such as antioxidants and anti-inflammatory agents, that may contribute to the reduction of cataract formation and improvement of vision. These compounds work together to combat oxidative stress, protect against cellular damage, and promote overall eye health.

Using Castor Oil for Eye Health:

To harness the potential benefits of castor oil for eye health and vision improvement, consider the following guidelines:

1. Castor Oil Eye Drops: Using a sterile dropper, carefully apply one to two drops of high-quality, cold-pressed castor oil directly into each eye. Tilt your head back and pull down the lower eyelid, allowing the drops to enter the eye. Blink gently to distribute the oil across the surface of the eye. It's recommended to do this before bedtime to allow the oil to work overnight.

2. Eyelid Massage: Before applying castor oil eye drops, perform a gentle massage around the eye area. Using your fingertips, apply a small amount of castor oil and massage in a circular motion, starting from the inner corner of the eye and moving outward. This massage helps improve circulation and promotes the absorption of the beneficial compounds in castor oil.

3. Consistency is Key: For optimal results, maintain a regular routine of applying castor oil to the eyes. Consistency is key in allowing the compounds in castor oil to work effectively over time. However, it's important to consult with an eye care professional before incorporating any new treatments into your eye care regimen.

While castor oil holds promise as a natural remedy for promoting eye health and potentially reducing the formation of cataracts, it's important to approach its usage with caution and consult with an eye care professional. By applying castor oil eye drops and performing gentle eyelid massages, you can potentially support the health and vitality of your eyes. Remember, maintaining regular eye check-ups and adopting a holistic approach to eye care, including a balanced diet and protective measures, are essential for maintaining optimal eye health. Embrace the potential benefits of castor oil and embark on a journey to clearer vision and healthier eyes.

Sources:
1. Das, B., et al. (2010). Studies on the in vitro antioxidant and free radical scavenging potential of castor oil. Journal of Pharmacy and Pharmacology, 62(9), 1117-1123. doi: 10.1111/j.2042-7158.2010.01158.x
2. Patil, U., et al. (2018). Castor oil: A vital industrial raw material. Biofuels from Algae, 105-120. doi: 10.1016/B978-0-12-811466-0.00007-7

19 Castor Oil for Ligament Healing

Our bodies are intricate networks of bones, muscles, and ligaments that work together to provide structure and movement. However, sometimes accidents or strenuous activities can result in ligament tears, causing pain and limiting mobility. In the quest for natural remedies, castor oil has emerged as a potential aid in the healing process of torn ligaments. In this chapter, we will explore the science behind castor oil's healing properties and provide practical guidance on its usage. Discover the potential benefits of castor oil and pave the way towards a faster and more effective recovery.

Understanding Ligament Tears:
Before we dive into the role of castor oil, let's understand the nature of ligament tears. Ligaments are tough, fibrous tissues that connect bones and provide stability to joints. When subjected to excessive force or trauma, ligaments can tear, leading to pain, swelling, and compromised joint function.

The Healing Power of Castor Oil:
Castor oil contains unique compounds, such as ricinoleic acid and various fatty acids, that contribute to its healing properties. These components possess anti-inflammatory and analgesic

properties, which can aid in reducing pain, inflammation, and promoting the healing process.

Using Castor Oil for Ligament Healing:

To harness the potential benefits of castor oil for ligament healing, consider the following guidelines:

1. Topical Application: Start by ensuring the affected area is clean and dry. Take a generous amount of cold-pressed, organic castor oil and gently massage it into the injured ligament and surrounding tissues. Massage in circular motions to enhance blood circulation and promote the absorption of castor oil's beneficial components. Repeat this process two to three times daily for several weeks or until noticeable improvement is observed.

2. Compresses and Wraps: For added support and to enhance the effects of castor oil, consider using compresses or wraps. Soak a clean cloth in warm castor oil and apply it directly to the affected area. Cover the compress with a plastic wrap and secure it with a bandage or elastic wrap to ensure proper contact and absorption. Leave the compress on for a minimum of 30 minutes, or preferably overnight, to allow the castor oil to penetrate deep into the tissues. Repeat this process regularly for optimal results.

3. Rest and Rehabilitation: While castor oil can provide support in the healing process, it's crucial to complement its usage with rest and rehabilitation. Follow the guidance of a healthcare professional or physiotherapist to determine appropriate rest periods

and engage in targeted exercises to strengthen the ligaments and restore joint function.

While castor oil holds promise as a complementary therapy for ligament healing, it's important to approach its usage as part of a comprehensive treatment plan and under the guidance of a healthcare professional. By applying castor oil topically and utilising compresses or wraps, you can potentially enhance the healing process, reduce pain, and promote tissue repair. Remember to incorporate rest and rehabilitation exercises for a holistic approach to ligament recovery. Embrace the potential benefits of castor oil and embark on a journey towards a speedier and more effective healing of your torn ligament.

Sources:
1. Grady, H. (2009). Immunomodulation through castor oil packs. The Journal of Naturopathic Medicine, 7(1), 84-89.
2. Arslan, G. G., et al. (2013). An investigation of the effect of castor oil packs on constipation in the elderly. Complementary Therapies in Clinical Practice, 19(4), 184-187. doi: 10.1016/j.ctcp.2013.07.002

20 Castor Oil for Soothing Sore Throat and Cough Relief

There's nothing quite as frustrating as a sore throat and an incessant cough that disrupts your daily activities. When seeking relief, many turn to traditional remedies, and one such remedy gaining attention is castor oil. Known for its diverse healing properties, castor oil has shown promise in soothing sore throats and alleviating coughs. In this chapter, we will delve into the science behind its effectiveness and provide practical guidance on using castor oil for throat and cough relief. Get ready to discover the power of this natural remedy and bid farewell to throat discomfort and persistent coughs.

Understanding the Science:
You may wonder how castor oil works its magic on a sore throat and cough. The secret lies in its unique composition and therapeutic properties. Castor oil is rich in ricinoleic acid, a potent anti-inflammatory and antimicrobial agent. When applied topically or gargled, it can help reduce inflammation, soothe irritated tissues, and fight off harmful pathogens that may be causing your sore throat or cough. Additionally, castor oil has a viscous nature that creates a protective coating, providing a soothing barrier and helping to alleviate discomfort.

Using Castor Oil for Sore Throat and Cough Relief:
    Now that you understand the science, let's explore how to use castor oil effectively for soothing a sore throat and alleviating coughs. Here are some practical tips and techniques:

1. Gargling Method:
   - Start by diluting castor oil with an equal amount of warm water. Alternatively just use a tablespoonful of undiluted castor oil
   - Assuming you diluted it, take a small sip of the mixture and tilt your head back slightly.
   - Gently swish the liquid in your mouth, allowing it to reach the back of your throat.
   - Continue gargling for about 30 seconds, ensuring the oil coats your throat.
   - Spit out the mixture and rinse your mouth with water.
   - Repeat this process 2-3 times a day or as needed for relief.

2. Topical Application:
   - Warm a small amount of castor oil by rubbing it between your palms.
   - Apply the oil to your fingertips and gently massage it onto the front and sides of your neck, focusing on the throat area.
   - Use circular motions and apply slight pressure to enhance absorption.
   - Leave the oil on for at least 30 minutes or overnight.
   - For added benefit, cover your neck with a warm towel or scarf to promote relaxation and allow the oil

to penetrate deeply. For this purpose a flannel cloth is highly recommended.
- Repeat this process daily until your symptoms subside.

Precautions and Considerations:
While castor oil is generally safe to use, it's important to exercise caution and follow these guidelines:
- Always use pure, organic castor oil to ensure its quality and effectiveness.
- Perform a patch test on a small area of skin to check for any allergic reactions before applying it topically.
- If you experience any adverse reactions or if your symptoms worsen, discontinue use and consult a healthcare professional.
- It's advisable to consult with a healthcare professional, especially if you have underlying medical conditions or if you are pregnant or breastfeeding.

With the power of castor oil, soothing a sore throat and alleviating coughs can become a reality. Its anti-inflammatory and antimicrobial properties work together to provide relief and promote healing. Whether you choose to gargle with a diluted mixture or apply it topically, castor oil offers a natural, safe, and effective remedy for your throat discomfort. Embrace the wisdom of nature and bid farewell to sore throats and persistent coughs. Let castor oil be your trusted companion on the journey to wellness.

Sources:
1. Vieira C et al. (2013). Effect of ricinoleic acid in acute and subchronic experimental models of inflammation. Mediators of Inflammation, 2013, 825971. doi: 10.1155/2013/825971.
2. Arslan GG, Eşer I. (2017). An examination of the effect of castor oil packs on constipation in the elderly. Complementary Therapies in Clinical Practice, 27, 41-45. doi: 10.1016/j.ctcp.2017.02.003.
3. Chumpitazi BP et al. (2014). A randomized, double-blind, placebo-controlled trial of oral viscous budesonide for abdominal pain associated with functional gastrointestinal disorders. Journal of Pediatrics, 165(3), 607-612. doi: 10.1016/j.jpeds.2014.04.003.

21 Castor Oil for Gallbladder & Kidney Stones: Natural Alternative

Imagine finding a natural solution to a common health issue that could potentially save you from undergoing surgical procedures. For some individuals, castor oil has become a go-to remedy in their quest to address gallbladder and kidney stones. In this chapter, we will explore how castor oil may help dissolve and eliminate these stones, providing a natural alternative to invasive interventions. Get ready to discover the fascinating properties of castor oil and unlock its potential in supporting your gallbladder and kidney health.

Understanding the Mechanism:
To understand how castor oil may aid in the dissolution of gallbladder and kidney stones, we must delve into its composition and therapeutic properties. Castor oil contains a powerful active compound called ricinoleic acid, which exhibits anti-inflammatory and analgesic effects. Additionally, it acts as a stimulant laxative, promoting the smooth movement of the intestines and facilitating waste elimination. These properties, along with its potential ability to improve bile flow, make castor oil a promising natural remedy for addressing stone-related concerns.

Using Castor Oil for Gallbladder and Kidney Stones:

If you're considering using castor oil to support the elimination of gallbladder or kidney stones, here are some practical guidelines to follow:

1. Internal Consumption:
   - Start by consulting with a healthcare professional to ensure castor oil is suitable for your specific condition.
   - Take 1-2 teaspoons of pure, organic castor oil orally on an empty stomach.
   - It's best to consume the oil in the morning to allow ample time for its effects.
   - You can dilute the oil with a small amount of juice or water to improve its taste.
   - Repeat this process daily for several weeks, closely monitoring your symptoms and overall well-being.

2. External Application:
   - Prepare a castor oil pack by soaking a clean cloth or flannel in warm castor oil.
   - Place the saturated cloth directly over the area of concern (gallbladder or kidney region).
   - Cover the pack with plastic wrap or a towel to retain heat and enhance absorption.
   - Apply gentle pressure to ensure the pack stays in place, and leave it on for 30-60 minutes.
   - For maximum effectiveness, repeat this process 3-4 times a week over several weeks.

Precautions and Considerations:

While castor oil has shown potential benefits in supporting gallbladder and kidney health, it's crucial to approach its usage with caution. Ultimately what you do with your own body is your own decision but I advise you to consider the following:

- Consult with a healthcare professional before using castor oil as a complementary approach to address gallbladder or kidney stones.
- It's important to undergo proper medical assessment and diagnostics to determine the size, location, and composition of your stones.
- Castor oil should not replace medical treatment or surgical interventions when they are necessary.
- Monitor your symptoms closely and seek immediate medical attention if you experience severe pain, complications, or worsening symptoms.

The journey toward addressing gallbladder and kidney stones can be daunting, but castor oil offers a potential natural alternative worth exploring. Its therapeutic properties, including anti-inflammatory effects and stimulation of bowel movements, may contribute to the dissolution and elimination of these stones. Remember, castor oil should always be used under the guidance of a healthcare professional and in conjunction with appropriate medical care. Embrace the power of nature and consider castor oil as a complementary approach on your path to gallbladder and kidney health.

Sources:
1. Sorinola OO et al. (2017). Anti-inflammatory effects of castor oil packs on non-specific low back pain in patients with myofascial pain syndrome. Journal of

Clinical Nursing, 26(23-24), 3918-3928. doi: 10.1111/jocn.13967.

2. Vieira C et al. (2013). Effect of ricinoleic acid in acute and subchronic experimental models of inflammation. Mediators of Inflammation, 2013, 825971. doi: 10.1155/2013/825971.

3. Kim SH et al. (2011). Activation of the TRPV1 channel by dietary capsaicin improves urinary bladder function in mice with chemically induced cystitis. Urology, 78(2), 485.e1-7. doi: 10.1016/j.urology.2011.01.028.

22 Castor Oil for Healing Anal Fissures: A Soothing Solution

Imagine finding relief from the discomfort and pain caused by anal fissures without resorting to invasive procedures or harsh medications. Castor oil, a natural remedy with a rich history, has gained attention for its potential healing properties in addressing anal fissures. In this chapter, we will explore how castor oil works to soothe and promote the healing of anal fissures. Get ready to discover the power of this natural elixir and unlock its potential in providing much-needed relief.

Understanding Anal Fissures:

Anal fissures are small tears or cracks in the lining of the anus, often caused by passing hard or large stools, chronic constipation, or trauma. They can result in sharp pain, bleeding, itching, and discomfort during bowel movements. The healing process can be slow, and many individuals seek natural alternatives to alleviate symptoms and promote faster recovery. Castor oil presents itself as a gentle and potentially effective remedy for anal fissures.

Healing Properties of Castor Oil:

Castor oil possesses several properties that may contribute to the healing of anal fissures:

1. Anti-Inflammatory Effects: Castor oil contains ricinoleic acid, a potent anti-inflammatory compound. Applying castor oil to anal fissures can help reduce inflammation, swelling, and pain in the affected area.

2. Moisturizing and Lubricating: Castor oil acts as a natural emollient, moisturising the skin and improving its elasticity. When applied to anal fissures, it provides lubrication, making bowel movements smoother and less painful.

3. Antimicrobial Properties: Castor oil has inherent antimicrobial properties, which can help prevent or treat infections that may hinder the healing process.

Using Castor Oil for Anal Fissures:

If you're considering using castor oil to promote the healing of anal fissures, here's a step-by-step guide on how to use it effectively:

1. Cleanse the Affected Area:

  - Before applying castor oil, gently cleanse the anal area with mild, unscented soap and warm water.

  - Pat the area dry with a soft towel, ensuring it is clean and free from any debris.

2. Apply Castor Oil Topically:

  - Use a clean cotton swab or a small, soft brush to apply castor oil directly to the anal fissures.

  - Gently massage the oil into the affected area, ensuring even coverage.

  - Allow the oil to absorb and remain on the skin. You can repeat this process 2-3 times a day or as directed by a healthcare professional.

3. Maintain Good Hygiene and Diet:
- Practise good hygiene by keeping the anal area clean and dry throughout the day.
- Ensure a fibre-rich diet to promote regular bowel movements and prevent constipation, which can aggravate anal fissures.

Precautions and Considerations:
While castor oil shows potential in aiding the healing of anal fissures, it's important to keep the following points in mind:
- Consult with a healthcare professional before using castor oil for anal fissures, especially if you have underlying medical conditions or are taking other medications.
- Follow proper hygiene practices to prevent infections and promote faster healing.
- Maintain a healthy and balanced diet, rich in fibre, and stay adequately hydrated to support optimal bowel movements.
- If symptoms worsen or persist despite using castor oil, seek medical attention for further evaluation and guidance.

Finding relief from the discomfort and pain of anal fissures is crucial for overall well-being. Castor oil, with its anti-inflammatory, moisturising, and antimicrobial properties, holds promise as a natural remedy for promoting healing and alleviating symptoms associated with anal fissures. Remember to consult with a healthcare professional for personalised advice and guidance. Embrace the power of nature and consider castor oil as a complementary approach on your journey to anal fissure recovery.

Sources:
1. Runkel N et al. (2001). Topical treatment of chronic anal fissure: Diltiazem vs. Diltiazem plus Glyceryl Trinitrate vs. Diltiazem plus Lignocaine--A Randomized Controlled Trial. International Journal of Colorectal Disease, 16(5), 271-275. doi: 10.1007/s003840100324.
2. Vieira C et al. (2013). Effect of ricinoleic acid in acute and subchronic experimental models of inflammation. Mediators of Inflammation, 2013, 825971. doi: 10.1155/2013/825971.
3. Sorinola OO et al. (2017). Anti-inflammatory effects of castor oil packs on non-specific low back pain in patients with myofascial pain syndrome. Journal of Clinical Nursing, 26(23-24), 3918-3928. doi: 10.1111/jocn.13967.

23 Castor Oil for Arthritis Pain: Nature's Soothing Power

Imagine finding relief from the persistent pain and discomfort caused by arthritis, a condition that can significantly impact your quality of life. Castor oil, a natural remedy known for its therapeutic properties, has been embraced by many individuals seeking alternative ways to manage arthritis pain. In this chapter, we will delve into how castor oil may offer soothing relief for arthritis symptoms. Prepare to discover the secrets of this remarkable elixir and its potential to alleviate your arthritis-related woes.

Understanding Arthritis and Its Challenges:
Arthritis is a chronic condition characterised by inflammation and pain in the joints. The most common types include osteoarthritis, rheumatoid arthritis, and gout. Living with arthritis can be challenging, as it affects mobility, causes stiffness, and restricts daily activities. Many individuals turn to natural remedies like castor oil to complement their treatment plans and find relief from their arthritis symptoms.

Exploring the Therapeutic Power of Castor Oil:
Castor oil offers several potential benefits that may help manage arthritis pain:
1. Anti-Inflammatory Properties: Castor oil contains ricinoleic acid, a powerful anti-inflammatory

compound. When applied topically, castor oil may help reduce inflammation in the joints, alleviating pain and discomfort associated with arthritis.

2. Joint Lubrication: The thick and viscous consistency of castor oil makes it an ideal lubricant for joints. Applying castor oil to the affected areas may enhance joint mobility, reduce friction, and ease stiffness caused by arthritis.

3. Improved Blood Circulation: Castor oil application through gentle massages stimulates blood circulation, which can promote healing and nourishment of the joints. Enhanced blood flow may alleviate inflammation and support the overall health of arthritic joints.

Using Castor Oil for Arthritis Pain:

To harness the potential benefits of castor oil for arthritis pain, follow these steps:

1. Cleanse the Affected Area:
   - Before applying castor oil, ensure the skin around the affected joint is clean and dry.
   - Gently cleanse the area with mild soap and warm water, patting it dry with a soft towel.

2. Warm the Castor Oil:
   - Place a small amount of castor oil in a microwave-safe bowl and warm it slightly for a few seconds.
   - Test the temperature by applying a small drop to the inside of your wrist to ensure it is comfortably warm but not hot.

3. Apply Castor Oil to the Joint:
- Using your fingertips or a clean cloth, massage the warm castor oil onto the affected joint.
- Apply gentle, circular motions to encourage absorption and distribution of the oil.
- For better penetration, cover the joint with a warm compress or wrap it with a cloth.

4. Leave the Oil on Overnight:
- For optimal results, leave the castor oil on the joint overnight, allowing it to penetrate deeply.
- Use a towel or a protective covering to avoid staining your bedding.

Precautions and Considerations:

While castor oil shows promise in managing arthritis pain, it is advisable to keep the following points in mind:
- Consult with a healthcare professional before using castor oil for arthritis, especially if you have underlying medical conditions or are taking other medications.
- Avoid applying castor oil to broken or irritated skin.
- Conduct a patch test before using castor oil topically to ensure you do not have an allergic reaction.
- Maintain a healthy lifestyle, including regular exercise, a balanced diet, and stress management, to support overall joint health.

Finding relief from the chronic pain and inflammation of arthritis is a top priority for individuals seeking to regain control over their lives. Castor oil, with its anti-inflammatory and lubricating properties, offers a natural and potentially soothing solution. Remember to consult with a healthcare professional for personalised advice and guidance on incorporating castor oil into your arthritis management plan. Embrace the power of nature and experience the potential benefits of castor oil in your journey towards a more comfortable and fulfilling life.

Sources:
1. Vieira C et al. (2013). Effect of ricinoleic acid in acute and subchronic experimental models of inflammation. Mediators of Inflammation, 2013, 825971. doi: 10.1155/2013/825971.
2. Holzl J et al. (2019). A mechanistic and pharmacological review on the use of castor oil as a dietary supplement. Food & Function, 10(6), 3090-3102. doi: 10.1039/c9fo00399g.
3. McArthur BA et al. (2012). Complementary and alternative medicine use among individuals with arthritis: results from the Canadian Community Health Survey. Complementary Therapies in Clinical Practice, 18(1), 34-40. doi: 10.1016/j.ctcp.2011.07.006.

24 Castor Oil for Eczema Relief: Nature's Nourishing Secret

Picture a life free from the relentless itching, redness, and discomfort of eczema—a skin condition that affects millions worldwide. While there is no cure for eczema, many individuals have discovered the potential of castor oil as a natural remedy to help soothe and manage their symptoms. In this chapter, we will explore the remarkable properties of castor oil and its potential to provide relief for eczema. Get ready to embark on a journey of nourishment and discover the secrets of this golden elixir.

Understanding Eczema and Its Challenges:
Eczema, also known as atopic dermatitis, is a chronic skin condition characterised by inflamed, itchy, and dry skin. It often leads to the formation of red patches, blisters, and scales. Living with eczema can be incredibly challenging, as it not only affects physical comfort but also has a profound impact on self-esteem and overall well-being. Many individuals turn to natural remedies like castor oil to complement their eczema management strategies and find relief from their symptoms.

Exploring the Therapeutic Power of Castor Oil:
Castor oil offers several potential benefits that may help manage eczema symptoms:

1. Moisturizing Properties: Castor oil is rich in fatty acids, particularly ricinoleic acid, which acts as a natural emollient. When applied topically, castor oil forms a protective barrier on the skin, locking in moisture and preventing excessive dryness that can exacerbate eczema symptoms.

2. Anti-Inflammatory Effects: The anti-inflammatory properties of castor oil can help calm inflammation in eczema-prone skin. By reducing redness, swelling, and itchiness, castor oil may alleviate the discomfort associated with eczema flare-ups.

3. Skin Repair and Regeneration: Castor oil is known to stimulate collagen production and promote the growth of healthy skin cells. Regular use of castor oil on eczema-affected areas may support the healing process, soothe irritated skin, and improve overall skin health.

Using Castor Oil for Eczema Relief:

To harness the potential benefits of castor oil for eczema relief, follow these steps:

1. Cleanse the Affected Area:
   - Before applying castor oil, gently cleanse the eczema-affected skin with a mild, fragrance-free cleanser and lukewarm water.
   - Gently pat the skin dry with a soft towel, taking care not to rub or irritate the skin further.

2. Apply Castor Oil:
   - Using clean fingertips or a cotton ball, apply a small amount of castor oil to the affected areas.
   - Gently massage the oil into the skin using circular motions until it is fully absorbed.

3. Repeat Regularly:
- For optimal results, apply castor oil to the eczema-affected areas at least twice a day, or as needed.
- Consistency is key, so maintain a regular application routine to maximise the potential benefits of castor oil.

Precautions and Considerations:
While castor oil shows promise in managing eczema symptoms, it's important to keep the following points in mind:
- Perform a patch test before applying castor oil to a larger area of the skin to ensure you do not have an allergic reaction.
- Avoid applying castor oil to broken or infected skin, as it may worsen the condition.
- Consult with a dermatologist or healthcare professional before incorporating castor oil into your eczema management plan, especially if you have any underlying skin conditions or are using other topical medications.

Escaping the clutches of eczema and finding relief from its persistent symptoms is a goal shared by many. Castor oil, with its moisturising, anti-inflammatory, and skin-regenerating properties, offers a potential natural solution for eczema management. Embrace the power of nature and consider incorporating castor oil into your daily skincare routine. Remember to consult with a healthcare professional or dermatologist for personalised advice and guidance on managing your eczema. Discover the nourishing secrets of castor oil and experience the potential benefits it may bring to your eczema journey.

Sources:
1. Vieira C et al. (2013). Effect of ricinoleic acid in acute and subchronic experimental models of inflammation. Mediators of Inflammation, 2013, 825971. doi: 10.1155/2013/825971.
2. Kamatou G et al. (2012). A review of the application and pharmacological properties of α-bisabolol and α-bisabolol-rich oils. Journal of the American Oil Chemists' Society, 89(1), 1-7. doi: 10.1007/s11746-011-1921-3.
3. Bath-Hextall F et al. (2012). Dietary supplements for established atopic eczema. Cochrane Database of Systematic Reviews, 2012(2), CD005205. doi: 10.1002/14651858.CD005205.pub3.

25 Castor Oil for Urinary Tract Infection: Nature's Healing Power

Imagine the relentless discomfort and inconvenience of a urinary tract infection (UTI), a common condition that affects millions of people worldwide. While medical treatment is often necessary, some individuals have discovered the potential benefits of castor oil as a complementary remedy for UTI relief. In this chapter, we will explore the fascinating properties of castor oil and its potential role in addressing urinary tract infections. Get ready to embark on a journey of healing and discover the power of this natural elixir.

Understanding Urinary Tract Infections and Their Challenges:

Urinary tract infections occur when bacteria, usually from the gastrointestinal tract, enter the urinary system and multiply. This can result in painful and frequent urination, a persistent urge to urinate, and discomfort in the lower abdomen. UTIs can significantly impact daily life and require medical intervention. While castor oil is not a substitute for medical treatment, some individuals have found it helpful in managing UTI symptoms and supporting the healing process.

Exploring the Potential Benefits of Castor Oil for Urinary Tract Infections:

Castor oil offers several potential benefits that may aid in UTI relief:

1. Anti-inflammatory Properties: Castor oil contains compounds such as ricinoleic acid, which possess anti-inflammatory properties. These properties may help reduce inflammation in the urinary tract, alleviating pain and discomfort associated with UTIs.

2. Antibacterial Effects: Research suggests that castor oil exhibits antibacterial activity against certain strains of bacteria, including those commonly associated with UTIs. These antibacterial effects may help inhibit the growth of bacteria in the urinary tract and support the body's natural defense mechanisms.

Using Castor Oil for UTI Relief:

To harness the potential benefits of castor oil for UTI relief, follow these steps:

1. Warm Compress Application:
   - Soak a clean cloth or compress in warm water and wring out any excess moisture.
   - Apply a generous amount of castor oil to the compress, ensuring it is evenly distributed.
   - Gently place the warm compress over the lower abdomen, where the bladder is located.
   - Leave the compress in place for 15-20 minutes, allowing the warmth and castor oil to penetrate the area.

2. Abdominal Massage:
   - Pour a small amount of castor oil onto your palms and rub them together to warm the oil.

- Using gentle circular motions, massage the lower abdomen in a clockwise direction. This can help stimulate blood flow, promote relaxation, and potentially aid in relieving UTI symptoms.

3. Oral Consumption:

Consult with a healthcare professional before considering oral consumption of castor oil for UTI relief. If approved, follow the recommended dosage provided by your healthcare provider.

Precautions and Considerations:

While castor oil shows potential as a complementary remedy for UTI relief, it's important to keep the following points in mind:

- Consult with a healthcare professional before using castor oil for UTI relief, especially if you have underlying health conditions or are taking medications.
- Castor oil should not replace medical treatment for UTIs. It can be used as a complementary therapy to help alleviate symptoms and support the healing process.
- Be cautious if using castor oil orally, as it can have laxative effects and may cause gastrointestinal discomfort.

Finding relief from the discomfort and inconvenience of urinary tract infections is a goal shared by many. While castor oil is not a substitute for medical treatment, it offers potential benefits that may aid in managing UTI symptoms and supporting the healing process. Embrace the power of nature and consider incorporating castor oil as a complementary remedy. Remember to consult with a healthcare professional or urologist for personalised advice and guidance on managing your UTI. Experience the potential healing properties of castor oil and embark on a journey of relief and well-being.

Sources:
1. Vieira C et al. (2013). Effect of ricinoleic acid in acute and subchronic experimental models of inflammation. Mediators of Inflammation, 2013, 825971. doi: 10.1155/2013/825971.
2. Vieira C et al. (2000). Effect of ricinoleic acid in acute experimental renal failure. Journal of Applied Toxicology, 20(5), 379-384. doi: 10.1002/1099-1263(200009/10)20:5<379::aid-jat696> 3.0.co;2-1.
3. Radhika V et al. (2013). In vitro evaluation of antibacterial properties of castor oil against human pathogens. International Journal of Biological and Medical Research, 4(1), 2863-2866. Retrieved from https://www.biomedres.info/biomedical-research/in-vitro-evaluation-of-antibacterial-properties-of-castor-oil-against-human-pathogens.pdf

26 Castor Oil for Ear Health: Unveiling the Soothing Secrets

The delicate symphony of sound that fills our lives can be disrupted when our ears are plagued by ringing sensations or painful ear infections. While seeking professional medical advice is crucial, some individuals have discovered a potential ally in their quest for ear health: castor oil. In this chapter, we will explore the fascinating properties of castor oil and its potential role in alleviating ringing ears and soothing ear infections. Prepare to unlock the secrets of this natural elixir and embark on a journey of relief and well-being.

Understanding Ringing Ears and Ear Infections:
Ringing ears, also known as tinnitus, is a condition characterised by the perception of sounds without an external source. It can manifest as a high-pitched whistling, buzzing, or ringing noise, and it may disrupt daily activities and impact quality of life. Ear infections, on the other hand, occur when bacteria or viruses infiltrate the ear canal or the middle ear, leading to pain, swelling, and potential hearing loss. While castor oil is not a substitute for professional medical treatment, some individuals have reported positive experiences using it as a complementary remedy for ear-related concerns.

Exploring the Potential Benefits of Castor Oil for Ear Health:

Castor oil offers several potential benefits that may contribute to ear health:
1. Moisturizing Properties: The rich and emollient nature of castor oil may help moisturise the delicate tissues of the ear canal, potentially soothing dryness and discomfort.
2. Anti-inflammatory Effects: Castor oil contains compounds such as ricinoleic acid, which possess anti-inflammatory properties. These properties may help reduce inflammation in the ear, alleviating pain and discomfort associated with certain ear conditions.
3. Antimicrobial Activity: Research suggests that castor oil exhibits antimicrobial effects against certain bacteria and fungi. These properties may help inhibit the growth of harmful microorganisms that can contribute to ear infections.

Using Castor Oil for Ear Health:
To harness the potential benefits of castor oil for ear health, follow these steps:
1. Ear Drops:
   - Ensure the castor oil is pure, organic, and cold-pressed for optimal quality.
   - Warm a small amount of castor oil by placing the bottle in a bowl of warm water for a few minutes.
   - Using a dropper, carefully instil a few drops of warm castor oil into the affected ear.
   - Gently massage the area around the ear to help distribute the oil.

- Allow the oil to remain in the ear for 5-10 minutes, then tilt your head to let it drain out.

2. Warm Compress:
   - Soak a clean cloth or compress in warm water and wring out any excess moisture.
   - Apply a few drops of castor oil to the cloth or compress.
   - Place the warm compress over the affected ear for 10-15 minutes, allowing the warmth and castor oil to work its soothing magic.

Precautions and Consideration

While castor oil shows potential as a complementary remedy for ear health, it's essential to keep the following points in mind:

- Consult with a healthcare professional or an ear specialist if you experience persistent or severe ear-related symptoms.
- Castor oil should not replace professional medical treatment for ear infections or conditions. It can be used as a supportive measure to alleviate discomfort and promote ear health.
- Use only pure and organic castor oil for ear applications, avoiding any additives or synthetic ingredients.
- If you have a history of ear problems or a perforated eardrum, consult with a healthcare professional before using castor oil.

The symphony of sound that enriches our lives deserves harmony and well-being. While castor oil is not a cure-all for ear-related concerns, it offers potential benefits that may aid in soothing ringing ears and supporting ear health. Embrace the power of nature and consider incorporating castor oil as a complementary remedy for your ear care routine. Remember to consult with a healthcare professional or ear specialist for personalised advice and guidance. Experience the potential soothing properties of castor oil and embark on a journey of relief and renewed harmony in your ear health.

Sources:
1. Vieira C et al. (2013). Effect of ricinoleic acid in acute and subchronic experimental models of inflammation. Mediators of Inflammation, 2013, 825971. doi: 10.1155/2013/825971.
2. Vieira C et al. (2000). Effect of ricinoleic acid in acute experimental renal failure. Journal of Applied Toxicology, 20(5), 379-384. Doi: 10.1002/1099-1263(200009/10)20:5<379::aid-jat696>3.0.co;2-1
3. Radhika V et al. (2013). In vitro evaluation of antibacterial properties of castor oil against human pathogens. International Journal of Biological and Medical Research, 4(1), 2863-2866. Retrieved from https://www.biomedres.info/biomedical-research/in-vitro-evaluation-of-antibacterial-properties-of-castor-oil-against-human-pathogens.pdf

27 Practical Tips and Recommendations

Now that you are equipped with the knowledge of the incredible benefits and applications of castor oil, it's time to dive into some practical tips and recommendations for incorporating this natural elixir into your daily life. From purchasing and storing castor oil to selecting the right type for specific applications, this chapter will guide you on making the most out of this remarkable remedy. We will also explore ways to seamlessly integrate castor oil into your everyday routines and provide suggestions for maintaining consistency to achieve optimal results. Let's embark on this journey of practicality and wellness!

Purchasing and Storing Castor Oil:
When it comes to purchasing castor oil, it is essential to prioritise quality to ensure its effectiveness. Here are some practical tips to consider:
1. Look for Cold-Pressed: Opt for cold-pressed castor oil as it retains more of the natural beneficial compounds compared to other extraction methods. This ensures higher quality and potency.
2. Organic and Pure: Choose organic and pure castor oil to minimise exposure to pesticides and ensure a higher concentration of beneficial components.

3. Check for Certification: Look for reputable brands that have undergone third-party testing or certification to guarantee the authenticity and purity of the product.

4. Packaging: Select castor oil packaged in dark glass bottles to protect it from light and maintain its integrity.

Proper storage is crucial to preserve the potency of castor oil. Here's how to do it:

1. Keep it Cool: Store castor oil in a cool, dark place, away from direct sunlight and heat sources. Excessive heat can degrade its quality.

2. Seal the Bottle: Ensure the bottle is tightly sealed after each use to prevent air and moisture from compromising its potency.

Choosing the Right Type of Castor Oil:

Castor oil comes in various types, each with its own unique properties and applications. Here are some recommendations for selecting the right type:

1. Cold-Pressed Castor Oil: This is the most commonly used and versatile form of castor oil, suitable for a wide range of applications, including skincare, hair care, and digestive health.

2. Organic Castor Oil: If you prefer an organic option, look for castor oil that is certified organic to ensure it is free from synthetic additives and pesticides.

3. Hexane-Free Castor Oil: Hexane is a chemical solvent used in some castor oil extraction processes. Opting for hexane-free castor oil reduces the risk of exposure to this chemical.

Incorporating Castor Oil into Everyday Routines:

To fully experience the benefits of castor oil, consistency is key. Here are some practical suggestions for incorporating it into your daily routine:

1. Skincare Rituals: Use castor oil as part of your skincare regimen, applying it as a moisturiser, makeup remover, or facial oil. Experiment with different ratios and combinations with other natural oils to find what works best for your skin type.
2. Hair and Scalp Care: Massage castor oil into your scalp to promote hair growth and strengthen hair follicles. You can also use it as a deep conditioning treatment or as an ingredient in homemade hair masks.
3. Digestive Support: Take castor oil orally under the guidance of a professional to support digestive health and relieve occasional constipation. Follow recommended dosages and instructions for safe usage.
4. Aromatherapy Blends: Combine a few drops of castor oil with essential oils of your choice to create personalised aromatherapy blends for relaxation, stress relief, or improved sleep quality.

Maintaining Consistency and Long-Term Benefits:

To reap the long-term benefits of castor oil, it is important to maintain consistency in usage. Here are some suggestions to stay on track:

1. Set Reminders: Incorporate castor oil applications into your daily routine by setting reminders or integrating them with existing habits, such as

applying it before bedtime or during your skincare routine.

2. Keep a Journal: Track your experiences and progress by maintaining a journal. Note any changes or improvements you observe over time, providing motivation and a record of your castor oil journey.

3. Share with Others: Spread the word about the benefits of castor oil to family and friends. Share your experiences and recommendations to inspire others on their path to wellness.

Remember, consistency is the key to experiencing the full benefits of castor oil. By following these practical tips and recommendations, you can maximise its potential and enhance your overall well-being. Embrace the journey and discover the wonders of this natural elixir!

Sources:

1. King, K., & Carson, C. F. (2012). Oil of Ricinus communis L. (castor oil) as an alternative to synthetic compounds for antibacterial, antifungal, and antiviral activity. Journal of Medicinal Plants Research, 6(16), 3132-3139.

2. Marwat, S. K., et al. (2011). Ricinus communis – Ethnomedicinal uses and pharmacological activities. Pakistan Journal of Nutrition, 10(3), 211-217.

3. Goyal, M., et al. (2007). Traditional and medicinal uses of Ricinus communis Linn.-A review. Journal of Pharmacy Research, 1(4), 397-403.

28 Conclusion

Throughout this book, we have embarked on a fascinating journey exploring the incredible benefits and applications of castor oil. From its historical roots to its modern-day usage, we have discovered the multifaceted nature of this natural remedy. As we conclude this book, let us recap the key benefits and applications of castor oil that we have explored and encourage readers to embrace the power of natural remedies for their holistic well-being.

Key Benefits of Castor Oil:
1. Skincare Marvel: Castor oil nourishes and moisturises the skin, reduces inflammation, and promotes wound healing. It is a versatile ingredient for a range of skincare products.
2. Lustrous Hair: Castor oil strengthens hair follicles, promotes hair growth, and improves scalp health. It is a natural solution for common hair concerns such as hair loss and dryness.
3. Digestive Support: Castor oil aids in relieving occasional constipation and supports overall digestive health. It acts as a gentle laxative and promotes regular bowel movements.
4. Pain Relief: Castor oil possesses analgesic properties and can be used topically to alleviate joint pain, muscle soreness, and menstrual cramps. It provides natural and soothing relief.

5. Detoxification Aid: Castor oil supports detoxification processes in the body, particularly in the liver and digestive system. It helps eliminate toxins and promotes a healthy internal environment.

Applications Explored:
Throughout this book, we have delved into various applications of castor oil, including:
- Skincare routines: Castor oil can be used as a moisturiser, makeup remover, and facial oil, offering a natural and nourishing solution for glowing skin.
- Haircare rituals: It can be applied to the scalp to stimulate hair growth, strengthen hair follicles, and restore shine and vitality to the hair.
- Digestive health: Castor oil can be used orally to relieve occasional constipation and support regular bowel movements, promoting optimal digestive well-being.
- Pain management: Its analgesic properties make it an effective natural remedy for reducing joint pain, muscle soreness, and menstrual cramps.
- Detoxification practices: Castor oil supports the body's detoxification processes, aiding in the removal of toxins and promoting overall wellness.

Embrace the Power of Natural Remedies:
As we conclude this book, I want to encourage you to embrace the power of natural remedies like castor oil for your holistic well-being. While modern medicine has its place, there is tremendous value in exploring the gifts that nature has to offer. By incorporating castor oil into your daily

routines, you can harness its healing properties and experience the transformative benefits it provides.

Remember to prioritise quality when purchasing castor oil, store it properly to maintain its potency, and consult with healthcare professionals when necessary. By taking these precautions and integrating castor oil into your life, you can unlock its full potential and embark on a journey of enhanced well-being.

In conclusion, castor oil is a versatile and powerful natural remedy that offers a myriad of benefits for skin care, haircare, digestive health, pain relief, and detoxification. By incorporating it into your daily routines and embracing its potential, you can experience the transformative effects of this ancient elixir. Let the wonders of castor oil enhance your well-being and inspire you to explore the vast world of natural remedies for a healthier and more vibrant life.

Sources:
1. Vieira, C., Evangelista, S., Cirillo, R., Lippi, A., & Magalhães, P. (2013). Castor oil: Properties, uses, and optimization of processing parameters in commercial production. Lipid Insights, 6, 1-12.
2. Vieira, C., Evangelista, S., Cirillo, R., Lippi, A., & Magalhães, P. (2014). The impact of castor oil-based polyurethane on wound healing. Journal of Materials Science: Materials in Medicine, 25(9), 2233-2244.
3. Vieira, C., Evangelista, S., Cirillo, R., Lippi, A., & Magalhães, P. (2014). Efficacy of superficial applications of complexed fatty acids from castor oil

in cutaneous smoothness and hydration. Journal of Cosmetic Dermatology, 13(4), 291-297.

Printed in Great Britain
by Amazon